# THE STATE OF THE
# PRISONS – 200 YEARS ON

# THE STATE OF THE
# PRISONS – 200 YEARS ON

EDITED  BY DICK  WHITFIELD
*For the Howard League*

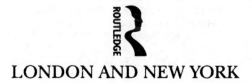

LONDON AND NEW YORK

First published in 1991
by Routledge
2 Park Square, Milton Park, Abingdon, Oxon, OX14 4RN

Simultaneously published in the USA and Canada
by Routledge
a division of Routledge, Taylor & Francis
270 Madison Ave, New York NY 10016

Transferred to Digital Printing 2006

Typeset by LaserScript Limited, Mitcham, Surrey

*British Library Cataloguing in Publication Data*
The state of the prisons – 200 years on.
1. Penal system, history
I. Whitfield, Dick G. (Richard George), *1939–*
II. Howard League for Penal Reform.
364.609

*Library of Congress Cataloguing in Publication Data*
The State of the prisons – 200 years on/edited by Dick Whitfield
for the Howard League.
p.  cm.
Includes bibliographical references and index.
1. Prisons – Cross-cultural studies. I. Whitfield, Dick, 1939–
II. Howard League for Penal Reform.
HV9443.S73   1990        90-39726
365 – dc20        CIP

ISBN 0-415-05187-8

Front Cover illustration: Mike Abrahams/Network
Front Cover design: Carole Oliver

**Publisher's Note**
The publisher has gone to great lengths to ensure the
quality of thisreprint but points out that some
imperfectionsin the original may be apparent

# CONTENTS

CONTENTS

# FIGURES AND TABLES

# THE CONTRIBUTORS

**Kevin Bales** is Senior Lecturer in Policy Studies at the Polytechnic of Central London, England. He has researched and worked on prison conditions and criminal justice in the United States with the Southern Coalition on Jails and Prisons.

**Ginny Baumann** is the Religious Group Adviser for Shelter, the national campaign for the homeless in Great Britain. She visited Nicaragua whilst acting as an Information Worker for Christian Aid.

**Norman Bishop** acts as an *ad hoc* expert at the Helsinki Institute for Crime Prevention, affiliated with the United Nations. He is the former head of the research and development group, Swedish Prison and Probation Administration.

**R.W. Burnham** is a criminologist and UK permanent representative with the United Nations at Vienna. His chapter was written whilst he was the George J. Beto Visiting Professor at the Sam Houston State University, Huntsville, Texas.

**Anton M. van Kalmthout** is Senior Lecturer in Criminal Law at the Catholic University of Brabant, Tilberg, Netherlands.

**Christian Kuhn** works in the Vienna Central Prison and represents the Howard League at the United Nations International Centre in Vienna, Austria.

**Dirk van der Landen** is Junior Lecturer in Criminal Law at the Catholic University of Brabant, Tilberg, Netherlands.

**Mike Maguire** is currently at the Department of Social and Administrative Studies, University of Wales, at Cardiff. His research was carried out whilst he was a member of the Centre for Criminological Research, University of Oxford, England.

THE CONTRIBUTORS

**Monika Platek** is an assistant professor at the Institute of Penal Law, Warsaw University, Poland.

**Andrew Rutherford** is Reader in Law at the University of Southampton, England, and Chair of the Howard League.

**Dirk van Zyl Smit** is an advocate of the Supreme Court of South Africa, Professor and Director of the Institute of Criminology, University of Cape Town 1982–9, and Dean of the Faculty of Law 1990.

**Brian Smith** is a lay magistrate who sits in the Nottingham Petty Sessional Division, England.

**Dick Whitfield** is Chief Probation Officer for the English county of Kent and Vice Chair of the Howard League.

# INTRODUCTION
*Penal reform and prison realities*
ANDREW RUTHERFORD

As to what is still wrong, I set down matter of fact without amplifi-
cation; which would in the end rather impede than promote the
object of my wishes; that is the corrections of what really is amiss.
The journeys were not undertaken for the traveller's amusement;
and the collections are not published for general entertainment;
but for the perusal of those who have it in their power to give
redress to the sufferers.

(Howard 1929)

Between 1773 and his death at Kherson in the Ukraine in 1790, John
Howard travelled, mostly on horseback, at least eighty thousand
kilometres, and probably a great deal further, as a self-appointed
inspector of prisons. While much of the journeying was in Britain
and Ireland, his half-dozen ventures abroad took him across much
of continental Europe. His method was simple and direct. He
visited, at considerable risk to his health, prisoners at their place of
confinement. Not for Howard the prison tour which, avoiding the
darker recesses, steered clear of the conditions endured by all those
confined. Howard's accounts received such widespread attention at
the time and are still read two hundred years after his death because
he so precisely 'set down matter of fact'. His general purpose was to
humanize prison conditions and to provide prisoners with opportunities for personal reformation. He became keenly aware that
there was much to be learned from practice overseas but his method
remained essentially descriptive, allowing his meticulously detailed
reports to speak for themselves. This volume is published as a tribute
to the genius and humanity (borrowing Edmund Burke's words) of
what remains the most exhaustive enquiry into prison conditions in
Europe. These essays on prisons across the world follow Howard's

1

descriptive method. Each addresses an individual prison and in most of them the author is either an 'outsider' or a foreigner, or both. Although the focus is on individual prisons, some account is taken of the wider prison system and, in at least some cases, the overall criminal justice process.

The most striking aspect of prison reform over the last two centuries is how little of it there has been. In most instances, the gains have been modest, tenuous and often short-lived. Even the more substantial changes pale against the broad sweep of political, social and economic progress over this period. There can be little doubt that John Howard, rising from his grave, would find much more that is familiar to him within the prison than across society as a whole. To enter the prison is, more often than not, to step back in time. In exploring why this should be, this introduction seeks to identify the choices for contemporary reformers.

The inherently authoritarian structure of the prison, deriving from its main functions of control and security, relies upon explicit threats of force which would be unacceptable elsewhere in a liberal democratic state. An American lawyer has graphically underlined this point by observing that the prison displays many features of the police state (Marin 1983: 75). It is this gap of values, arising from the use of imprisonment in a free society, that largely sets the prison reform agenda. That reformers are often frustrated testifies to the reality of what prison is about. As a former minister of justice in Sweden remarked, 'I do not mean that it is wrong to "humanize" the stay in prison – but a cage is still a cage, even if gold-plated' (Ward 1979). Winston Churchill, that most remarkable of Home Secretaries, summed up the point with characteristic eloquence:

> We must not allow optimism or hope or benevolence in these matters to carry us too far. We must not forget that when every material improvement has been effected in prisons, when the temperature has been rightly adjusted, when the proper food to maintain health and strength has been given, when the doctors, chaplains and prison visitors have come and gone, the convict stands deprived of everything that a free man calls life. We must not forget that all these improvements, which are sometimes salves to our consciences, do not change that position.
>
> (House of Commons 1910)

As associated reality is the regressive character of prison conditions.

For every step forward, the institution often seems to slip back two steps. John Howard, acutely aware of such slippage, argued that good staff and external vigilance were essential if reform efforts were to be sustained, but this view, as we look back over the last two centuries, may have been unduly optimistic. A less sanguine conclusion was reached by Jerome Miller, who for two years attempted to transform the young offender institutions of Massachusetts into therapeutic communities before coming convinced that the only appropriate course of action was to empty them. Miller observed that penal institutions 'cannot sustain their decency over an extended period of time. They tend ultimately to move towards repression and violence at worse, and apathy at best. And apathy is ultimately violence' (Rutherford 1986: 72). This regressive phenomenon has also been highlighted by Her Majesty's Chief Inspector of Prisons in a report on Feltham Youth Custody Centre. For many years, Feltham had sought to engage staff constructively with especially challenging and often mentally disordered young men. The Home Office decided to rebuild the institution, at a cost that exceeded £25 million. The 'new generation' prison architecture promised small living units and close involvement of staff. The inspector, however, found that any bonuses deriving from this design 'have been lost and also much of the experience and skill of the "old Feltham" which coped well with a difficult borstal population'. The opening sentence set the report's tone. 'It seems particularly unfortunate to find within the elegant and modern buildings of Feltham, so carefully landscaped, all the defects of poor regimes' (Home Office 1989). Even though there were some special local problems to take into account, to a large extent the regime at Feltham, where teenagers spent most of their time locked up in their cells, was victim to the malaise endemic to the prison system as a whole.

In 1926 Fenner Brockway, who had been imprisoned during the First World War, wrote in a newspaper article: 'The object of penal reformers should not be to reform the prison system but to abolish it' (Priestley 1988: 175).

Brockway was writing in the context of a prison population for England and Wales that had declined by two-thirds over the previous fifty years. This assertion is important for two main reasons. Firstly, the endorsement of penal as distinct from prison reform implied that the target for change had shifted from the prison to the

3

criminal justice process as a whole. The need for a wider focus had been signalled five years earlier when the merger of the Howard Association and the Prison Reform League resulted in the establishment of the Howard League for Penal Reform. Prisons, it was being insisted, should not be regarded in isolation from the wider picture. To do so was to invite disappointment if not disaster. Before pursuing this theme, attention should be directed at the other issue arising from Brockway's declaration, the abolitionist stance, which eschews efforts to improve life within prisons in favour of seeking to be entirely rid of the prison system. Later abolitionists, most notably Thomas Mathiesen, have argued that only 'negative' reforms (changes that may reduce the debit side of the prison's legitimacy but add nothing to the credit side) be encouraged. By contrast, 'positive' reforms (changes that improve the system so that it works more effectively) should be resisted (Mathiesen 1984). The abolitionist stand does provide a warning beacon against which penal policies, such as prison building programmes, might be assessed. Less radical than the abolitionist, but perhaps more realistic, the reductionist seeks a minimalist prison system (which it might be argued England, with a rate of 28 prisoners per 100,000 inhabitants, was not far from at the time of Brockway's article) within which reasonably decent standards might be maintained.

## THE PENAL TRINITY

Any realistic attempt to improve prison conditions must take full account of two pivotal aspects of the prison system, namely population and capacity. Indeed, the inter-connections of this penal trinity of population, capacity and conditions form the heart of the reform quagmire.

Massive prison population expansion in recent years is by no means unique to the United States, but it would be difficult to find other examples where during the 1980s the annual rate of growth exceeded 11 per cent. Between 1950 and 1989 the total number of people held in gaols and prisons across the United States leapt from 264,500 to 999,400.[1] In 1989 the rate of prisoners per 100,000 inhabitants was 422, considerably in excess, as reported in this volume, of the rates for South Africa (373) and Poland (177). For England and Wales, this has also been a period of considerable growth, with the prison population more than doubling between

4

1950 and 1980, from 20,400 to 50,000. In September 1988, for the first time, Britain led the Council of Europe table with rates for England and Wales and for Scotland of 97 and 99 per 100,000 respectively (Council of Europe 1988). The profound consequences of escalating numbers of this kind reach across the country; an ever-widening circle of people is touched by, if not directly caught up within, the prison system. No predictable relationship exists between prison population and the level of recorded crime, and disproportionately large prison populations scar the landscape of any state with pretensions to liberal values. Furthermore, expanding prison populations have crippling consequences for prison regimes. Pressure of numbers impinges on every facet of the prison system, and in some institutions has resulted in overcrowded conditions that would not have been tolerated a century earlier. Not least has been the impact upon staff, often reduced to a warehousing role in conditions of acute stress.

Building new prisons is often presented in terms of reform. John Howard's proposals for a national penitentiary, R.A. Butler's building programme announced in his 1959 white paper, *Penal Practice in a Changing Society*, and the contemporary notion of the 'new generation prison' have each, in their own time, promised a new dawn. In England and Wales, France and the United States huge prison building programmes were underway during the 1980s. A fairly modest plan in England, announced in 1980, had by 1989 been expanded to 25,000 new places, an increase, at a cost of £1,000 m., of almost 60 per cent in total capacity by the mid-1990s. At first there was support for this construction from some liberal quarters, encouraged by the government's commitment to 'eliminate' overcrowding. However, the vehement opposition to prison building by penal reform groups appears to have been vindicated in the light of a worsening of overcrowding and the further deterioration of regimes. While in France there were signs of a reassessment of the building programme (which was reduced in the late 1980s from 15,000 to 13,000 new places) the expansion in the United States has continued unabated. Between 1978 and 1985 some 165,000 new prison places were created and extensive additions are planned for the remainder of the century. There is the danger that new prison space may prompt additions to the prison population. While such Parkinsonian notion has an attractive simplicity it has so far eluded empirical verification (see Blumstein, Cohen and Gooding, 1983,

5

for the refutation of one such claim), it is clear that under certain circumstances capacity may act as a brake on population expansion. The mechanism of the 'waiting list' worked in this way in The Netherlands during the twenty-five years up to 1975 (Rutherford 1986) and the logic of rationing scarce custodial space is at the heart of the Minnesota Sentencing Guidelines Commission. The Guide-lines Commission interpreted an ambiguous statutory injunction that it take correctional resources into 'substantial consideration' as a mandate that its guide-lines not increase prison population beyond existing capacity constraints (Tonry 1988). Although it appears that sentencing became more severe during the first three years the guide-lines were in use, Minnesota remains one of the very few states that has avoided huge increases in prison population size (Parent 1988).

Far from leading to improved conditions, building new prisons may often have the contrary result. In part, the high-cost squalor that characterizes many expansionist prison systems results from a trade-off between capacity and conditions with respect to the allo-cation of public finances. Pumping much of the enhanced capital expenditure into new prison building often has the effect of drain-ing the prison of vital resources. Nor does the intention of building in order to replace obsolete prisons tend to work out in practice. In reality, the new prison is built and the old prison remains.

Not all efforts to improve prison conditions are futile, but any success is likely to be at the margins and will depend upon full regard being given to the capacity and population side of the reform equation. Some progress can, in these circumstances, be made to reduce what David Downes has called the 'depth of imprisonment' (Downes 1988). On the basis of interviews with prisoners in The Netherlands and England, Downes concluded that there was less 'depth' to imprisonment in the former, a parallel to John Howard's conclusion two centuries earlier: 'I do not know which to admire most, the neatness and cleanliness appearing in the prisons, the industry and regular conduct of the prisoners, or the humanity and attention of the magistrates and regents.' Much, however, remains elusive about the quality of life within prison, as was observed in a study which found a generally negative impact on prison regimes in England resulting from 'Fresh Start', the new staff working arrange-ments (King and McDermott 1989).

If the primary object of penal reformers is not to abolish prisons it is certainly to secure reductions in prison population. The starting-point is to recognize that the size and composition of the prison system, far from somehow being predetermined, are the consequence of action taken at every stage of the criminal justice process. Practitioners, to a very large degree, hold the keys to reform. Much depends upon their feeling empowered to reverse expansionist trends. While a great deal depends upon reform efforts outside the prison system (and indeed these efforts are often located outside the criminal justice process), prison personnel do not have to play the passive roles in which they tend to be cast.

## REFORM FROM WITHIN

Shining examples of prisons as decent and constructive places generally are brief episodes, often associated with particular staff members who display a combination of exceptional vision, determination and charisma. Within larger prison systems, such regimes can, at best, usually be counted in single numbers. The names of certain prison governors whose personal positive qualities permeated every aspect of their prisons tend to be long remembered. Most such British lists would probably include Alan Roberton, David Hewlings and Bill Perrie. In the United States, Frank Wood, the Warden of Oak Park Heights prison in Minnesota, comes to mind, as, in Denmark, does Erik Anderson. While it is not suggested that this roll of honour is exhaustive, a list would, even on a world-wide basis, be strikingly short. It is notable that in the prisons featured in this book, the head of prison emerges, if at all, as an anonymous official. In some instances the stride forward is restricted to one section, often quite small, of the prison. The special unit at Barlinnie Prison, near Edinburgh, which opened in 1973, is especially well known. For this eight-bed unit, the inspirational force was a senior prison officer, Ken Murray. However, Murray left the Scottish prison service prematurely and the problem is always one of whether such pioneering work can be sustained or indeed survive much change.[2]

Much of the impetus for improving conditions within the prison and for creating a regime that is built upon mutual respect between staff and prisoners depends upon initiatives taken by prison staff. Aspects of this process are described in a remarkable essay by Michael Jenkins, written just before his departure as Governor from

7

Long Lartin Prison. That an ethos of this kind exists at Long Lartin has, since the time of its first Governor, Bill Perrie, been widely recognized, and it is one of only two top security prisons to avoid serious control problems. Jenkins argues that

> the prison system has a tendency to create more problems than it receives and has an equal tendency to fail inmates because, out of its survival fear, it tends to respond to corporate threats, real or imaginary, rather than the real problems of inmates.
>
> (Jenkins 1987)

Of crucial importance is an 'unwritten contract' between staff and prisoners, the primary function of which is 'to get people sensibly through their sentences' (Jenkins 1987: 270). Jenkins believes that 'we can genuinely offer prisoners more than an antidote to the deterioration they fear' and that a regime is possible that engenders 'hope and optimism' (1987: 277).

However, the prison and the system of which it is part tend to resist internal reform initiatives. Occasional collective efforts by prisoners to improve their lot have mostly been sharply put down. The events associated with the prisoners' rights movement that flourished for a time in the late 1960s and early 1970s in parts of the United States, Scandinavia and Britain had by the early 1980s largely disappeared without trace. The authoritarian and mechanistic character of the prison system also ensures that the staff reformer is vulnerable to being co-opted, marginalized or driven out. Very occasionally, reformers are found in the higher reaches of the system, but in these instances their effectiveness tends to be compromised and their occupancy of top positions short-lived. Among the few notable and recent examples of reforming leadership within prison systems, mention might be made of H.H. Brydensholt in Denmark, Hans Tulkens in The Netherlands, Ken Schoen in Minnesota and, with respect to youth prison systems, Jerome Miller in Massachusetts.

To be effective, the internal prison reformer has to reach out and encompass not only conditions but the related issues of capacity and population. The connections between these three issues need to be kept in mind, although opportunities for the internal reformer to make them effectively will greatly vary. Internal reformers need to be in contact with like-minded people located across the criminal justice process and in particular with persons making decisions

8

about the use of custody. This means they must actively encourage a more selective approach to custodial remand and sentencing. They must also endorse an openness and frankness about conditions within the prison and the likely negative impact of the experience of imprisonment. It almost certainly means they must counter those forces within the prison system which have a vested interest in expansion. How, for example, can a debate be generated within expansionist prison systems about the merits of seeking additional funds for capital expenditure? Certainly, in essence this is a political decision, but it would be naïve to play down the extent to which this and other aspects of the policy agenda is shaped by officials. Internal prison reformers cannot divorce themselves from these issues, however sensitive they might be. There is also the associated and delicate issue of contact between internal reformers and reforming pressure groups. Such contacts are likely to be discouraged if not banned by the system and will necessarily need to be handled with the utmost discretion.

Reforming officials within both the prison system and the criminal justice process cannot afford to be merely reactive. A pro-active stance is essential in terms of setting and maintaining the mood for change across the various agencies of justice. That such a mood, primarily among prosecutors, judges and defence lawyers, has been a critical feature of the recent decline in the prison population of the Federal Republic of Germany is now well established (Feest 1988, Rutherford 1988). What professionals discuss informally at conferences and on other occasions, within and across agency lines, is as important as contributions to journals in setting and sustaining this mood. Recent explorations of the roots of Dutch reductionist penal policy highlighted the distinctive influence of the Law Faculty at Utrecht University for a generation of criminal justice practitioners. An intermingling of policy makers, practitioners and academics created an anti-penal ambience that continues to pervade the Dutch penal scene. Juvenile justice practice across much of England and Wales during the 1980s has displayed somewhat similar features (Rutherford 1989). Criminal justice practitioners need also to be proactive on the wider public stage. According to David Downes, Dutch elites have 'a distinct appreciation of the extent to which community tolerance cannot be taken for granted, but needs active elicitation and encouragement'. He goes on to observe that

9

the roots of reductionism seem to drive not so much from a free-floating tolerance on the part of the people in general but from the convictions of the most influential elites that crime is best combated by social and institutional, rather than specifically penal means.

(Downes 1988)

Many efforts by practitioners to achieve criminal justice reform are based upon adaptations, alterations and additions to the formal structure. An example of the prosecution stage in England is the Public Interest Discontinuance project initiated by the Vera Institute of Justice in 1988, in close co-operation with the Crown Prosecution Service and the Inner London Probation Service. By providing the prosecutor with additional information about the defendant, the scheme seeks, in appropriate cases, to suggest alternatives to prosecution. At the bail stage, the Vera Institute has also been active on a number of fronts. The Bail Information Schemes being developed in England and Wales also provide the prosecutor with additional information that might reduce requests for custodial remands. It is at the sentencing stage where formal strategies are most often to be found. Examples range from efforts to structure sentencing decisions through legislative criteria (for example, Criminal Justice Acts 1982 and 1988) to the far-reaching Minnesota Sentencing Guidelines Commission. Guidelines methods are also to be found at later decision-making stages of the process, governing, for example, emergency release, temporary release and parole practice (Gottfredson 1987). Structural reform by itself, however, is unlikely to deliver the required change of direction and it is certainly not a substitute for the commitment of inside reformers to shape policy and practice.

We should, perhaps, not be surprised that such modest progress has been made in improving prison conditions since John Howard's time. Prison reformers have been slow to adapt to prison realities, and to accept that they must address the wider canvas of the criminal justice process. The reductionist position is that, within a system spared down to minimal size, prisons can sometimes, at least for a while, be made reasonably decent places. But this state of affairs can be achieved not only by people working within the prison system, but by activating and empowering a much wider spectrum of practitioners.

## NOTES

1 Personal communication from the Bureau of Justice Statistics, United States Department of Justice, September 1989.
2 Curiously, two recent accounts of the Barlinnie Special Unit make no mention of Murray. See Coyle (1987) and Whatmore (1987) in A.E. Bottoms and R. Light (eds) *Problems of Long-Term Imprisonment*, Aldershot: Gower, but see also Jimmy Boyle (1977) *A Sense of Freedom*, London: Pan.

## REFERENCES

Blumstein, A., Cohen, J. and Gooding, W. (1983) 'The influence of capacity on prison population: a critical review of some recent evidence', *Crime and Delinquency* 29: 1–51.

Council of Europe (1988) *Prison Information Bulletin* 12, Strasbourg: Council of Europe.

Downes, D. (1988) *Contrasts in Tolerance, Post-war Penal Policy in The Netherlands and England and Wales*, Oxford: Oxford University Press.

Feest, J. (1988) *Reducing the Prison Population: Lessons from the West German Experience?*, London: National Association for the Care and Resettlement of Offenders.

Gottfredson, D. (1987) 'The problem of crowding: a system out of control', in S.D. Gottfredson and S. McConville, *America's Correctional Crisis*, New York: Greenwood Press.

Home Office (1989) *H.M. Young Offenders Institution and Remand Centre, Feltham, Report by H.M. Chief Inspector of Prisons*, London: HMSO.

House of Commons (1910) Debates: 5th Series, Vol. 19, London, columns 1353–4.

Howard, J. (1929) *The State of the Prisons*, London: J.M. Dent.

Jenkins, M. (1987) 'Control problems in dispersals', in A.E. Bottoms and R. Light (eds) *Problems of Long-Term Imprisonment*, Aldershot: Gower, 261–80.

King, R.D. and McDermott, K. (1989) 'British prisons 1970–1987, the ever-deepening crisis', *British Journal of Criminology* 29: 107–28.

Marin, B. (1983) *Inside Justice: A Comparative Analysis of Practices and Procedures for the Determination of Offences Against Discipline*, London: Associated University Press.

Mathiesen, T. (1984) *The Politics of Abolition*, Oxford: Martin Robertson.

Parent, D. (1988) *Structuring Criminal Sentences, The Evolution of Minnesota's Sentencing Guidelines*, Stoneham, Massachusetts: Butterworths Legal Publishers.

Priestley, P. (1988) *Jail Journeys*, London: Routledge: 175.

Rutherford, A. (1986) *Growing Out of Crime*, Harmondsworth: Penguin.

—— (1988) 'The English penal crisis: paradox and possibilities', in R. Rideout and J. Jowell (eds) *Current Legal Problems*, London: Stevens, 93–113.

—— (1989) 'The mood and temper of penal policy, curious happenings in England during the 1980s', *Youth and Policy* 27: 27–31.

Tonry, M. (1988) *Structuring Sentencing*, in M. Tonry and N. Morris (eds) *Crime and Justice, A Review of Research*, Chicago: University of Chicago Press.

Ward, D.A. (1979) 'Sweden: The Middle Road to Prison Reform' in M.E. Wolfgang (ed.) *Prisons, Present and Possible*, Lexington, Massachusetts: Lexington.

# Chapter One

# MAIDSTONE PRISON, ENGLAND

## *DICK WHITFIELD*

I

John Howard visited Maidstone Prison twice. By the time of his first visit in 1779, there had been a county gaol in the town for over two centuries but although the building he visited was only thirty-three years old he was very critical of the facilities it provided. The original prison, inconveniently situated in the High Street, was small, over-crowded, without an exercise yard and incapable of expansion. Yet the 'new' prison which Howard visited was equally poor. The small, mean courtyards meant a lack of light or air and despite the use of a sail ventilator to remedy the poor air circulation, Howard foresaw further problems.

Without great attention to cleanliness and the separation of the sick, he warned, there was a great danger of gaol fever. The 'awful, contagious disorder' struck in 1783 and killed twenty prisoners and a carpenter who was working in the gaol. Despite remedial work, which Howard acknowledged on a second visit in 1786, the prison was clearly still inadequate.

Finally, in 1806, the West Kent justices conceded that the prison would have to be completely rebuilt. Daniel Alexander, the architect of Dartmoor Prison, was appointed and it was decided that the new building should be constructed on the lines recommended by Howard: individual sleeping cells for prisoners, with day-rooms, courtyards and offices: a strict separation of different classes of prisoner and careful attention to problems of water supply, sewerage and ventilation. The architect, having toured a number of prisons, reported to the justices: 'In the gaol I have endeavoured to adopt, after much pains and meditation, the good parts of every gaol I have visited, preferring, I own, the principle of Ipswich by

Blackburn, Howard's disciple' (Melling 1969: 208).[1]

Alexander's new gaol remains the nucleus of Maidstone Prison today. It was completed in 1819 at what was then the staggering cost of £163,457 and was the largest and most imposing building in the town. Nineteenth-century prints show how it dominated the skyline and the area around. Now, offices, the County Hall and even a car park make a bigger impact but the prison retains its huge central site. Solid and secret behind a high stone wall it remains a world apart from the crawling traffic which skirts it on the routes out of town.

## II

Probably the most overworked word in any description of the British prison system over the last decade or more has been 'crisis'. A crisis of inmate unrest, with recurrent rooftop protests or rioting; a staff crisis, with the Prison Officers' Union forcing thousands of prisoners to be held in police cells; above all, a numbers crisis, with successive Home Secretaries announcing, at various times, that the breaking point of the system would be reached when the prison population passed the 40,000, or the 44,000, or the 50,000 mark. Throughout this time, prison staff and managers passed the various 'crisis' totals, got on with the task, absorbed everyone sent to them by the courts and, somehow, despite a crumbling prison estate, avoided total chaos.

The reason for this inexorable rise in numbers lies in the use of imprisonment by British courts both before and after trial. In simple numbers the annual average prison population has grown as shown in Table 1.1. Within these figures there have been peaks as high as 51,000, necessitating the short-term use of military camps to contain the new army of prisoners. The proportion of those on remand, that is, being held prior to trial or sentence, was 14.5 per cent in 1979 but in 1988 had grown to 23 per cent, with the average waiting time for trial at the Crown Court also increasing.

Some of those held on remand will be found not guilty and a significant proportion do not receive custodial sentences when their case is finally heard – points not lost on the government, which is investing in additional bail hostels, special bail information schemes run by the probation service and, more controversially, pilot schemes making use of electronic 'tagging' equipment; these are all

*Table 1.1* Average daily prison population, England and Wales

| | |
|---|---|
| 1979 | 42,220 |
| 1980 | 43,109 |
| 1981 | 43,436 |
| 1982 | 43,754 |
| 1983 | 43,773 |
| 1984 | 43,349 |
| 1985 | 46,278 |
| 1986 | 46,889 |
| 1987 | 48,963 |
| 1988 | 49,900 |
| 1989 | 48,610 |

*Sources:* Home Office (1987) *Prison Statistics, England and Wales,* London: HMSO
Home Office (1990) *Statistical Bulletin 12/90,* London: HMSO

ways, it is hoped, to reduce what many see as an unnecessary and wasteful use of prison resources.

An equal problem is created by trends in sentencing. Between 1983 and 1988 the number of men serving short sentences (defined in Britain as 18 months or less) fell by 27 per cent. In the same period the number of men serving medium sentences (18 months to 4 years) rose by 34 per cent and of long sentences (4 years or more) by no less than 82 per cent. The sheer length of sentences imposed, especially when contrasted with our European neighbours, presents enormous management problems in prisons, as the description of Maidstone Prison will show. Beneath these lengthening sentence trends, however, are other equally disturbing problems. Twenty years ago, only 10 per cent of the prison population was aged under 21 years. The proportion now is 33 per cent. Similarly, ethnic minorities are disproportionately represented in prison. The figure had reached 15 per cent of the prison population by 1988 and Afro-Caribbean and African men seem to be most at risk. A belated but growing recognition of both of these problems has seen the development of some special initiatives designed to relieve them; it is too early to tell whether sentencing trends can be reversed but there are early indicators with the under-21s, who are being especially targeted by the probation service in offering courts non-custodial options, that are encouraging.

In comparative terms, Britain's use of imprisonment as a sanction remains high (Table 1.2) and current statistical projections on its continued use remain uniformly gloomy.

*Table 1.2* Prisoners per 100,000 population on 1 September 1988

| | |
|---|---|
| United Kingdom | 97.4 |
| Germany | 84.9 |
| France | 81.1 |
| Italy | 60.4 |
| Sweden | 56.0 |
| Norway | 48.4 |
| Holland | 48.4 |

*Source:* NACRO (1990) *Information Bulletin no. 25* (January), London:
National Association for the Care and Resettlement of Offenders

Every year, the Home Office, as the government department responsible for prisons, publishes two sets of projections for long-term trends in the prison population. The 'non-demographic' (NDM) projections only take account of expected trends in crime and the numbers sent to prison; the 'demographic' (DM) projections also take into account expected changes in the age structure of the general population. The main change is likely to be a fall in the number of young people, which ought to be reflected in the prison population. These projections give a prison population in 1997 of between 64,000 (DM) and 67,100 (NDM) – an increase of between 28 per cent and 34 per cent on current figures (Home Office 1989a).

It is a scenario which drew the following comment from the minister responsible:

For over a hundred years, penal policy in this country has appeared to focus on custody. If a fine is not enough, custody is said to be the only adequate penalty. Other orders are described as non-custodial penalties and assessed as alternatives to custody. All this reinforces custody in a central position. Why do we do this? I hope one of the outcomes of the debate will be to move the focus of penal policy away from custody. Let us think rather of a twin track approach, in which custody is reserved for those who commit serious offences. It should not be the final sanction to which all persistent criminals progress, however minor their offences. It will be a long haul, but we want to make out of date the notion that the only punishment that works is behind bars.

(The Home Secretary, quoted in NACRO Annual Report, November 1988)

The cost, in both human and financial terms, has been high. The prisons budget of £775 million in 1988 was set to rise by 42 per cent to £1,140 million in 1989, to cover the cost of expanding the prison building programme, emergency measures on overcrowding and the costs of keeping prisoners in police cells. It is a rate of growth no other public service could match. In human terms, the results of Britain's reliance on custody are soberly recorded in the annual reports of the Chief Inspector of Prisons. His report for 1988 concluded that 'in prison after prison men were still having to exist in conditions which offend against any standard of decency', and he remarked, 'Properly fitting clean clothes and regular baths or showers are not luxuries but they remained out of reach for many inmates in 1988' (Home Office 1989b).

On training prisons such as Maidstone he found, generally, that most establishments were struggling to provide a basic level of regime activities. He thought the quality of life for such prisoners was generally reasonable in that there was 'no deliberate neglect, no conscious inhumanity and no wilful omissions. The defects that existed in regimes resulted generally from staff shortages, concentration on other priorities, lack of good management or, at worst, lack of concern' (Home Office 1989b).

The response by government has – primarily – been to embark on a massive prison building programme, despite hopes of making the Home Secretary's 'twin-track' approach more of a reality. The building programme, the largest undertaken this century, provides for the construction of 26 new prisons between 1983 and 1995, at a total cost of £870 million at current prices. Together with a programme of expansion and refurbishment at existing prisons there will be an additional capacity of 21,000 places. In terms of relieving overcrowding and dealing with the decay of older prisons, new and refurbished buildings clearly have something to offer but the sheer scale and cost of the proposals (an average capital cost per place of £69,000 and thereafter £13,000 per prisoner per year to run) has drawn much critical comment.

This, then, is the backcloth against which Maidstone prison needs to be considered. Within the broad overall picture, built up from the 129 Prison Department establishments in England and Wales, Maidstone occupies a distinctive and significant place. Adult prisons (for those aged 21 or over) are divided into 'local' prisons, which receive people from the courts, whether on remand or at the start of a sentence (and where short sentences may be served in their entirety); closed 'training' prisons of which Maidstone is one, and 'open' prisons, which have a minimum of security and are for prisoners perceived as posing no real risk to the public. The main problems of overcrowding are in local prisons, which act as holding centres before inmates are moved to training or open prisons. But even closed prisons vary greatly, from the very high security (Category 'A') dispersal units to lesser security categories 'B' and 'C'. Maidstone, behind its high stone wall, is a Category 'B' prison.

## III

The first impression of any visitor to Maidstone prison must surely be one of confusion. The five and a half hectare site contains an astonishing jumble of over fifty separate buildings, ranging from the solid stonework of the 1819 prison to Victorian brickwork and a bewildering variety of modern additions, including the kitchens. There are four main residential blocks, or 'wings' with single cell accommodation; Medway, which takes 171 men, Kent (166), Weald (99) and Thanet (102). There is also a Segregation Unit, used both for punishment and to isolate men for their own protection or for other reasons; a hospital unit, and a hostel from which eleven men can work in the town during the day, returning to the prison each night. The prison's capacity, or certified normal accommodation (CNA), is 550.

In some ways, however, Maidstone is several small prisons within one perimeter, for in addition to being a training prison it has two special functions. The first, in Thanet wing, is to act as one of three Vulnerable Prisoner Units in the country. This is a national resource and prisoners are sent here who staff believe would be at risk of violence (because of their offence) in a normal prison setting, or whose fear of violence has led them, themselves, to request such a transfer. Many will have committed sexual offences that other prisoners find abhorrent; some will have been informers who helped the police in the hope of obtaining a shorter sentence and still others may have built up debts inside prison that they cannot repay. It means Thanet wing has to be a 'sterile' area, with staff at Maidstone always conscious of the need to keep its occupants separate from the rest of the prison or – when contact is inevitable – well controlled. At the time of my visit about half the men had been convicted of heterosexual offences, mostly rape; about a quarter for offences against children and about a quarter were the 'grasses' or informers. Thanet wing attracts additional staff to Maidstone Prison, especially for the Psychology Department, of which more will be said later. It ought to be able to offer more psychological and psychiatric help to the men who inhabit its strange, grey world; more group work as well as individual help is acknowledged as being required by the staff, including the Probation Officer, who have a special responsibility for it, for these are men for whom the risk of reconviction is often very high. Thanet wing, however, has as its primary purpose to keep its inmates from physical harm; the good work that is undoubtedly done there with individuals is almost a bonus.

All men at Maidstone are long sentence prisoners, serving more than four years, and it is at the top end of the scale, with life sentence prisoners, that Maidstone performs its second specialist task. Maidstone is one of a number of designated prisons able to take 'lifers' and it can provide up to 100 places for them, although there were only 80 at the time of my visit. Most are concentrated on Medway wing, but not all, and there is no sense of a special regime so far as they are concerned. The growing number of life sentence prisoners has been a considerable problem for the prison service for some years now. Life imprisonment is the mandatory sentence for murder but it is also the maximum sentence for a number of other offences, including manslaughter, armed robbery, wounding with intent, arson, rape, kidnapping, and causing an explosion. In 1957 there were just 140 lifers in prison; thirty years later, in 1987 the number had grown to over 2,200, of whom about one in five had received their life sentence for an offence other than murder.

The life sentence is indeterminate and although the average length of time served is just over ten years, many men stay in prison for much longer periods. Maidstone Prison contains one man who has already served 33 years and staff seemed torn between two beliefs; one, that the risk he posed (of further offences against children) meant that further incarceration was inevitable, the other that his extraordinarily long period in custody meant he would be unable to survive outside the prison walls, anyway. Not all life sentence prisoners follow the same 'career path' through prison but most spend three to four years in two initial centres, then progress to training prisons and – possibly – open prisons before a final release date is in sight. By the time they arrive at Maidstone, therefore, most have settled into the routines imposed by a long sentence of imprisonment and most do at least feel that some progress through the system is being achieved.

The life sentence prisoners are not the only ones serving long sentences; Maidstone also contained 133 men serving sentences of 10 years or more when I visited. For all kinds of prisoner, however, the daily routine is the same:

| | |
|---|---|
| 07.45 | Cells unlocked |
| 08.15 | Breakfast |
| 08.45 | Work starts |
| 11.15 | Exercise period |
| 11.45 | Lunch (in the dining room or in cells) |
| 12.00 | Prisoners again locked in cells |
| 13.30 | Cells unlocked |
| 13.45 | Return to work |
| or 14.00 | Visits for those who have visitors that day |
| or 14.00 | Use of sports area for those working on the wing |
| 16.15 | Work ends |
| 16.30 | Evening meal |
| 16.45 | Prisoners locked in cells |
| 17.45 | Cells unlocked for evening association, classes, television or church |
| 20.00 | Prisoners return to cells; locked up for the night |

The weekend routine varies, with no work to occupy the day and with extended exercise periods available to those who wish to use them. Exercise is, in fact, well provided for, with an indoor swimming pool, a gymnasium, a sports area for football (with teams from outside the prison involved in both football and weightlifting), and like most long-term prisons, Maidstone has its share of those who keep fanatically fit.

Work plays a large part as the centrepiece of the daily regime and both its opportunities and its shortcomings were made clear to me. The prison offers a mixture of straight employment and trade training courses, together with the many jobs which are essential to the daily running of an institution: cleaners, cooks, maintenance parties for both the buildings and the grounds. The work opportunities are primarily in the tailors' shop, a laundry (which services a number of other prisons), a printing shop and an assembly shop. The last is not fully operational yet; the hope is to undertake a wide range of light assembly work on outside contracts. But the men themselves, who call it 'the muppet shop', remain unconvinced that it really has anything to offer. 'It's just a form of brain death', said one lifer scornfully, and indeed for many men the repetitive, soul-destroying nature of much of the work would indeed seem only to add to the pains of imprisonment.

There is also a book-binding shop and a Braille Unit, which transfers a wide range of books into braille for the blind, and which really does serve a useful purpose. The notice-board in the work-room contains heartfelt letters of thanks from those who have received their new books and it is clear that the sense of involvement in the lives of real and unfortunate people in the outside world draws a very positive response from the men involved. I watched a man working on a special cookery book for a mother who is both blind and diabetic; he made it so obvious that he valued the opportunity to make some reparation that I wonder whether more opportunities like this could not be created.

The printing shop is, in many ways, typical of prison industry. It operates mostly on labour-intensive, repetitive government forms rather than the wider variety of commercial printing work which would give men a marketable skill on release as well as a good work experience. The civilian in charge was philosophical about this and recognized the limitations. 'We're just about to have a new camera and darkroom', he said, 'and then we shall only be about ten years behind the times.' Until more interesting work was available he felt he had no option but to keep the men in his charge fully occupied and if it meant using eight men to undertake a task which could be accomplished in a fraction of the time by a machine, well – the men weren't going anywhere.

Much more popular with the prisoners are the range of Vocational Training Courses (VTCs) which take men for a period of 20 or 26 weeks, give them a thorough training in a particular skill and enable them to take outside examinations. The certificates they obtain do not specify the centre as Maidstone Prison; they can be safely shown to employers and are much prized. At present, courses are run in bricklaying, painting and decorating, welding, and sheet metal fabrication, and as far as I could see the standard of work was generally very high indeed. The bricklaying course has some interchange with a local college and the prison instructor, surrounded by test pieces his charges had made (ornate archways, window frames and decorative walls) took pride in recalling that the prison 'pupils' often outshone their free counterparts.

The major frustration for prisoners is that these courses are so much in demand. Waiting lists of 80 or 100 men, many from outside Maidstone Prison, are commonplace. Prisoners made it clear that, from their point of view, ready access to such courses is one of the major improvements they would seek. The Governor and his staff have long recognized this and plans for two new courses, one in arts and crafts, the other on computers, are planned to start in 1990. They will go at least some way to removing the bottleneck.

For their work, prisoners receive minimal sums – between £2.20 and £4.60 per week, depending on the work and the hours involved. At the bottom end of the scale are the cleaners and those in full-time education; the printing shop pays £3.60 per week and the kitchen staff earn most, in recognition of the seven-day working week required.

Food, of course, remains a topic of passionate concern – the focus of minor complaints and disagreements which rumble on for long periods – and outbursts of contentment which are extremely short-lived. Most men seemed to find both the quantity and the variety quite acceptable and to recognize that, with a large institution and central kitchens, the variable quality was only to be expected. The very substantial meat pie, with vegetables (followed by sponge pudding and custard) that I saw served on Weald wing drew generally favourable comment. 'Well, perhaps the presentation could be improved' was the wry comment of one prisoner. Discontent seems to be centred more on those on special diets and, with vegetarians, vegans, Hindus, Muslims and Jews to cater for there is clearly scope for problems. To some extent this has been ameliorated by providing cookers on each of the wings. This enables men either to buy small stocks of supplies from the canteen with their earnings in order to cook for themselves, or to re-cook prison food in new and exciting ways. This has become something of an art form, with some prisoners acquiring an enviable reputation for transforming prison fare into spicy and original ethnic dishes. With up to 30 per cent of prisoners coming from minority backgrounds (mostly black and Asian, but with Polish, Irish and other groups also represented) this is one way of allowing for – and even valuing – cultural diversity and may be one reason why racial tensions do not seem to be as evident as one might expect. There is a much higher concentration of minority groups in Kent wing, together with a mosque and synagogue and it may be that this also helps.

So far, I have concentrated on some of the standard aspects of prison life and routine – in some ways no more than a mirror image of other large institutions. As an American writer observed recently, 'It was hard to distinguish hotels in England from prisons or hospitals. Most were run with the same indifference or cruelty and were equally uncomfortable' (Theroux 1984).

There are other features of prison life, however, which could only occur in this especially artificial environment, but before moving on to them it may be useful to concentrate on some of the prisoners' own views of Maidstone. I was allowed to disrupt a 'social skills' course – one of a number of educational opportunities for men apart from the usual classes – and took the opportunity to test out some of my impressions against their own, well-informed ones in a session that, in the end, lasted twice as long as its scheduled time.

Some of their views came as something of a surprise. Maidstone Prison has embarked on a long and costly process to bring integral sanitation to cells, to avoid the 'slopping out' process and the need to have chamber pots in cells. Prisoners were scornful about the sense of priorities this demonstrated, and about the supposed benefits. A system which allowed electronic unlocking of cells so that they could use shared toilet facilities seemed preferable to most. In any case they were quite clear where their own priorities lay:

1   *The availability of telephones* came easily top of the list. At present special requests have to be submitted and justified if calls are to be made; they are made in the presence of an officer and they are charged at far in excess of the 'normal' rate because of the need to ask the operator to ring back with the cost – for which a surcharge is made. Freer use of the telephone is being extended to prisons with a lesser security category; men in Maidstone cannot believe it would jeopardize security there if it were available.

2   *Better access to trade training courses.* One of the few ways that prisoners can feel that some positive benefit has been gained from a sentence.

3   *A fairer 'canteen' system:* The current system (which the Governor acknowledged was unsatisfactory) is particularly resented because prices are often higher than at other prisons, let alone

outside shops. Men feel exploited ('We earn less and pay more') and their inability to change things exacerbates the position they are in.

4 *Better education opportunities:* There was a general sense of dissatisfaction with education provision which seemed to relate more to whether it met people's needs than the actual range of classes provided. There were also acknowledged strengths, of which the Social Skills course was one. This took the place of a pre-release course (which would be impossible to plan in an institution where some men were so far away from release and others might be released on parole licence at very short notice) but it covered many of the same topics. Overseen by two prison officers with help from the Psychology Department, it runs for two weeks, full time on perhaps ten or twelve occasions per year. It uses outside speakers from the Social Security office, the Job Centre, and the Citizens' Advice Bureau and covers a wide range of current affairs and other topics in a relaxed and friendly way. Men use video cameras and produce and film 'news bulletins' as a useful way of learning to work in small groups, to see how they present themselves and to gain confidence generally. A similar special course, known as the 'Summer School', runs for life sentence prisoners and also tries to stimulate interest and enjoyment in equal measure.

All these are part of what might be termed the 'quality of life' and the prisoners' preoccupation with this vital but ill-defined subject is shared by the Governor, Graham Gregory-Smith.

Rehabilitation is not a real term for staff [he said], especially when men are serving such long sentences. Keeping them alive in mind and body is a much more accurate description of what we do. Prisoners have a genuine fear of becoming cabbages. Sustaining men through a long sentence is much more than providing work or classes, important though they are. Prisoners have to start getting used to *talking* to staff here, to making some of their own decisions and to finding out how Maidstone is different.

He agreed that the prison had a long-standing reputation of having a liberal regime and added, 'I would have been mad to try and change it radically. Altering it at the fringes and working hard on prisoner/staff relationships was much more what was needed.'

The springboard for these changes was 'Fresh Start', a concerted move in the prison service to change working practices, deployment of staff and work patterns; to move towards local accountability and control and to deal with industrial relations problems which otherwise looked to be endemic. Prison officers are now salaried and take time off in lieu rather than accumulate high earnings on overtime; they can purchase their own houses, and they can be promoted to governor grades rather than remaining a secondary uniformed branch. As the Governor observed, it takes more time to change attitudes, but he thought that progress was being made here too and that the new recruitment would accelerate the process.

Above all, 'Fresh Start' has encouraged the use of shared casework schemes in which prison officers and probation officers share work concerning prisoners much more effectively. The probation service's task in prison is primarily to provide a social work service to those imprisoned and there has always been a conflict between the day-to-day, mundane but pressing needs of prisoners cut off from family and friends, and the more reflective analytical and purposeful work related to offending behaviour in which Probation Officers wanted to engage. Maidstone now has a 'casework officer' scheme in which each prisoner has a particular officer on the wing to whom he can relate, as well as the services of the wing Probation Officer. Sharing work, yet retaining a clear sense of role, is obviously more difficult but potentially rewarding and in Maidstone seems to be working well. For the Governor, though, the main benefit has been that it gives prison officers 'permission to be concerned' in a structured and consistent way. Job status and job satisfaction, for most officers, is significantly improved.

There are eight governor grades and 174 uniformed staff at Maidstone. Add specialist and administrative staff, from clerks to teachers, to instructors and Probation Officers and the total is about one hundred higher. Only two of the current prison service staff are female, a fact much regretted by the Governor, who believes that up to 20 per cent of female staff would be beneficial in terms of that elusive 'quality of life' inside. Two groups of specialist staff have a particular role to play in this same area – psychologists and Probation Officers.

There should be five psychologists and one assistant at Maidstone Prison, but recruiting difficulties mean that two psychologist posts are vacant at present. Although based in Maidstone, they also have to provide a service to other prisons in the area and the problems posed by the over-stretching of this resource means that there is a limited impact on the prison. Much of the Psychology Department's work is concerned with research and management issues and their computer-based inmate data base is central to this. The department monitors the inmate population, offences against prison rules and the penalties awarded; it assists management in determining security grades and in assessments on life sentence prisoners; and it has been looking at the structures of meetings, the effectiveness of communications and the problems of stress in staff. Clinical work with prisoners depends partly on demand and partly on the willingness of psychologists to undertake it, for none are trained as clinical specialists. Nevertheless some valued individual work is undertaken and I was told it was often most effective when carried out jointly with a Probation Officer, each undertaking specific but complementary work.

The Probation Department has four Probation Officers and a Senior Probation Officer to provide a service to the prison. Although very much part of the probation service generally they are operationally responsible to the Governor for their period of secondment to the prison and this uncomfortable structural position – with one foot each side of the prison wall – brings both problems and opportunities. 'It's hard', said one Probation Officer; 'we're not actually part of anything and have to operate in a sort of no man's land.' Work with individuals can capitalize on not being part of 'the system', however, and from their offices on the wing the Probation Officers have easy and direct access both to prisoners and to other staff with whom they work. With long-term prisoners and lifers much of their work is centred on the understanding of offending behaviour and the risks of re-offending; with others, the whole range of family and personal problems call for tact, understanding and a good deal of dogged, patient work. 'Knowing when prisoners are *ready* to respond is the skill you learn to develop here', said one; 'the staff are a good lot and there is a positive culture in which to work – but you still have to work out when real work is possible and it's not just meeting institutional demands.'

The major frustration, for prisoners even more than Probation Officers, is the parole system. All the men on determinate sentences at Maidstone are eligible for parole, theoretically when one third of their sentence has been served. It is 'theoretically', because the then

Home Secretary introduced new guide-lines some years ago which severely restricted the application of parole to men serving sentences for offences of violence, sexual offences and the supply of illegal drugs. Henceforward these prisoners could be routinely *considered* (and the process is long, costly and complex, involving interviews, a local review board and then the national Parole Board) but would only be released before almost the end of their sentence in very exceptional circumstances. The result, for a man serving a twelve-year sentence in one of the new categories, would be that parole review at the four, five and six year mark would be a hollow charade. Even at the seven year mark there would be very little expectation of more than a few weeks on parole licence in the community, instead of prison. The potential gain if one was 'exceptional', however, and qualified for an early release is so powerful that few men are prepared to forego it. The result is a shabby, futile process that Probation Officers feel makes subsequent work with inmates more difficult; that exasperates prison officers who see the time and energy in compiling reports as wasted, and infuriates prisoners for whom the probable refusal of parole, with its tiny element of uncertainty, makes prison life even harder to bear. The problem is compounded at present by the bureaucracy of parole, which results in decisions being anything up to six or eight months late. Yet, overall, parole has been a substantial success in terms of successful supervision in the community. The complex arguments which lay behind the present situation – and the possible solutions – are, however, beyond the scope of this chapter. I can only record that prisoners and prison staff displayed a rare unanimity in condemning the present system.

IV

How can a complex institution like a prison be judged? My task was to record it as objectively as possible and leave the reader to judge, yet not to provide some indication of the effect it had on me would be to paint a very incomplete picture. Maidstone has the kind of problems which beset most prisons; illegal brewing remains a constant problem in which the ingenuity of prisoners is constantly pitted against the watchfulness of staff and the balance shifts constantly. Over 1,300 litres of highly alcoholic brew had been seized from one wing alone, in nine months. Drugs are equally problematic and with 'open' visits are almost impossible to contain. (Most prisoners come from the Greater London area, so family visits are relatively easy; a liberal visiting policy also means that up to three visits can be made during a month.) The attitude of wing prison officers to drugs was interesting. 'It's almost always cannabis', I was told, 'and I suppose if the Governor really wanted it stopped, he could – or near enough. But at what cost? It would mean searches on every visit, more restrictions, more repression and it would work against everything else we are trying to do. If it's manageable and doesn't get out of hand I reckon we accept it.'

There are problems, too, in the way in which different prisons have come to deal with long-term prisoners. This means some men transfer from Category 'A' prisons and find new rules at Maidstone which they believe are petty and restrictive, and facilities which seem less than those they enjoyed elsewhere, in supposedly stricter regimes. (Some were used to having freezers and food storage facilities as well as cookers on the wing and this restriction on individual choice, in a system where it is precious, hit hard.) Yet others, especially from the London prisons, found it relaxed, humane and positive. It all depends on their starting-point.

I suppose my starting-point was a phrase in a national newspaper, the *Sunday Times*, some years ago. Reviewing Britain's prisons, the paper summed them up as 'a decent sort of warehouse, doing its best not to let the stock deteriorate'. Given the pressures of numbers, limited resources for positive work in education and trade training, limited work opportunities and staff and prisoner unrest, even that modest aim has often seemed unattainable. Staff and prisoners at Maidstone were acutely aware that, in a training prison, they were relatively well off compared to the overcrowded local prisons, whose barren regimes often mean prisoners being locked in their cells twenty-three hours each day. Both groups seemed equally aware that they had a joint investment in making it work, for all its faults, as well as possible. In my view they do so with commitment and humanity. Who and how many people we imprison, for how long and in what conditions are questions that politicians and sentencers must answer; those in the prisons must make it work as well as they can. In Maidstone, they do.

## NOTE

1   Quoted in Melling, E. (ed.) (1969) *Crime and Punishment, Kentish Sources*, published by Kent County Council. For a fuller description of Howard's visits and proposals, see *The State of the Prisons in England and Wales*, 4th edn 1792, reprinted 1973, Montclair, NJ: Patterson, Smith.

## REFERENCES

Home Office (1989a) *Home Office Statistical Bulletin 11/89*, Croydon: Home Office Statistical Department.
Home Office (1989b) *Report of HM Chief Inspector of Prisons 1988*, London: HMSO.
Theroux, P. (1984) *The Kingdom by the Sea*, Harmondsworth: Penguin.

# Chapter Two

# THE INDIAN PRISON

## *MIKE MAGUIRE*

My starting-point was a search for details about 'conditions in a typical Indian gaol'. Despite problems of access, I gathered sufficient information about the physical conditions and regime in a particular central gaol to produce at least a poor imitation of John Howard. However, it soon became clear that, not only are Indian gaols so varied that to describe any one is to create a false picture, but a description of 'conditions' alone would give readers outside India little real insight into the country's prison system or how it is experienced by inmates. To achieve such insight, it is essential to understand something of the social and historical context.

There will be space here only for the briefest discussion of external forces which have shaped life in Indian prisons, but it is difficult to overestimate their importance. These include the 'legacy of the British', who promoted an overtly punitive penal philosophy, more concerned with the repression of dissent than with ordinary crime, and who ran the prisons as cheaply as possible; a labyrinthine criminal justice system, which causes many accused persons to spend years in gaol before their trial is completed; widespread political interference with the police, whereby criminals with 'connections' often escape justice, leaving the gaols populated predominantly with poor rural labourers; the designation of prisons, under the Seventh Schedule of the Constitution, as primarily the responsibility of the thirty-one individual states and union territories rather than the Indian government – which has perpetuated gross differences in practices and standards; and the generally low priority attached to 'non-productive' areas like penal reform in a country with 250 million people below the poverty line, where economic development dominates planning and expenditure.

In the following pages, I shall first present a broad picture of the Indian prison population and the institutions in which it is held. This is followed by some general remarks about the history and philosophy of imprisonment in India, and a summary of previous writers' conclusions about gaol conditions. I shall then describe conditions in the central gaol I visited, ending with some comments about the possibilities and prospects for change.

I

The convicted prison population in India is remarkably small. In a country of around 800 million, with over one and a half million police officers and nearly 1,200 gaols (not to mention a Draconian penal code drafted by the British in 1860), only about 60,000 people are serving sentences of imprisonment at any one time. In relation to population, this is five to ten times fewer prisoners than in European countries.

Sadly, though, the gaols do not stand half-empty. Convicted prisoners are outnumbered by the euphemistically named 'under-trials' – remanded prisoners for most of whom trial is months (if not years) away and many of whom, detained pending police investigations, have not yet been charged with an offence (Diaz 1977). In recent years, the officially recorded – and probably under-recorded – number of undertrials has frequently exceeded 90,000.

There are other categories of prisoner, too, smaller in number but whose presence raises serious questions about human rights. 'Detenus' – people held without trial under various Acts sanctioning preventive detention[1] – have sometimes attracted international concern, particularly during periods of internal tension when allegations of torture have accompanied protests about the detention of political prisoners.[2] But when the number of detenus returns to a more 'normal' level of 400–500, consisting mainly of suspected drug smugglers and 'dacoits'[3] rather than political activists, interest tends to fade.

'Non-criminal lunatics' and 'criminal lunatics' (the continued use of archaic terminology betraying attitudes towards them[4]) officially numbered 2,077 and 318, respectively, at the end of 1980, according to figures collected for the All-India Committee on Jail Reforms (1983). However, only half the states produced any statis-

31

tics, it not being standard practice to record lunatics as part of the prison population. (*The Punjab Jail Manual* (1975: 345) even states specifically that 'Non-criminal lunatics shall be entirely excluded from all statistical returns relating to jails.') If the figures produced by the state of West Bengal, which show non-criminal lunatics making up one in eight of its prison population, are a better guide to the true situation, the picture is grim indeed. Non-criminal lunatics, as the name implies, have committed no offence, but are people designated by a magistrate as 'wandering and dangerous lunatics' under the Indian Lunacy Act 1912 and sent to prison to await transfer to a mental hospital. As there are fewer than fifty such hospitals in the whole country, with long waiting lists and high proportions of permanent inmates, the '6 to 8 months' average waiting time reported by Guha (quoted in Baxi 1982) for a gaol in Assam may be shorter than the national average. Meanwhile, where 'criminal lunatics' are concerned, the All-India Committee (1983: para 3.24) produced the finding that 'Some have stayed in prison for more than 20 years without their trial even having begun.'

While the mentally ill remain very much part of the prison scene, the central government has recently taken action (Juvenile Justice Act 1986) to exclude another group who should certainly not be incarcerated. For many years, both prison reformers and official reports regularly condemned the presence of children in gaols, some below the age of 10. Many were homeless or orphaned, held in gaol owing to a lack of children's homes; others, it was even alleged, were deliberately arrested on flimsy pretexts to be exploited as unpaid servants or sweepers when the gaol population rose. Kuldip Nayar, a journalist detained during the Emergency, described the practice in Delhi's Tihar gaol thus:

> Even more shocking than the corruption was the ingenious 'slave system' we found in the jail. The slaves were boys between ten and eighteen employed as 'helpers', and there were scores of them . . . They would be woken up before 6 a.m. to prepare the morning tea and would be allowed to sleep around 10 p.m. . . . . They were herded into a ward which had no fan and no proper sanitary facilities . . .
>
> These boys were undertrial prisoners; many had been there for eight months and at least one had been there for two years. They were taken from one court to another to be tried under one

charge or another and kept in jail all the while. The aim was to keep them in as long as possible, for without them the people employed to do the menial duties would have no time to relax . . .

One morning I was woken by the sobbing of a boy . . . I asked him what he had done to land himself in jail. He was too racked by sobs to reply, but . . . the warder explained that whenever the number of prisoners in jail went up, the police were asked to bring in boys to help with the chores. For the past several days, the warder said, jail authorities had been pestering the police to get more helpers. . . . The evening before, when the boy was buying a betel-leaf from a shop, the police had hauled him up as a vagabond; they were responding to the jail authorities' appeal to book more helpers. . . . It was unbelievable that this could happen in the 20th century.

(Nayar 1978: 33)

While there is no evidence of such practices being widespread in the country, the fact that it could happen in the main prison in the capital of India was a matter of scandal. Moreover, even as late as 1985, an unpublished government document reveals, there were 989 children[5] among one day's population in Indian prisons, on 30 June 1985. According to criminologists I consulted, doubts remain whether the Act has entirely remedied the situation (magistrates and police are not always meticulous in determining offenders' ages), but it has certainly alleviated it considerably.

Finally, another category of prisoners – those held in 'protective custody' – has been greatly reduced in size recently, partly by the Juvenile Justice Act and partly as a result of the case of *Hussainara Khatoon* v. *Bihar* 1979, which declared their detention unconstitutional. Some of these were vagrant children, others victims of crime required as witnesses. In the *Hussainara* case, it was revealed that a number of destitute women had been held in prison for several years awaiting the trials of men accused of raping them.

Convicted prisoners, undertrials, detenus and 'lunatics', together with civil prisoners and various other small groups, make up an unknown total population in Indian gaols. Prison statistics are poor in quality and, like crime statistics, are published several years late. According to government officials I consulted, the prison population has settled down since 1977 (the end of the Emergency) in the range 150,000 to 180,000. However, this refers only to undertrials and convicts. Allowing for the categories omitted (not to mention possible undercounting in some of the slackly administered sub-gaols),[6] the true total could be several thousand higher.

For a breakdown of the characteristics of the prison population at any one time, one of the few available sources is the statistics collected for the All-India Committee on Jail Reforms 1980–3. These describe the population in all Indian gaols on 31 December 1980.

To Western eyes, the composition of the convicted population appears extraordinary (see Table 2.1). Over 40 per cent were serving life sentences for murder, while at the same time, almost as many were serving very short sentences. The extent of the turnover of short-termers is illustrated by statistics showing receptions into prison, as opposed to daily population. For example, Datir (1978: 212) found that, in the state of Maharastra, over two-thirds of all admissions of convicts to prisons were of people serving one month or less; and a third of admissions were for ticketless travel on the railway, usually through inability to pay fines.

By contrast, the type of prisoner most familiar in European and North American prisons, the habitual property offender serving a short- to medium-term sentence, is a comparative rarity in India. Among the total convicted population at the end of 1980, only 11 per cent were 'burglars' and 10 per cent 'thieves'. Around three-quarters of all convicts were first offenders.

There is a higher proportion of people from poor rural backgrounds in prisons than in the general population. Around half are illiterate. Indian prisoners are also generally older than prisoners in many other countries. A quarter of convicts are over 40 (Table 2.1), mainly because of the exceptionally long periods that 'lifers' spend in gaol: the minimum period to be served is fourteen years.

The available information about undertrials is rather less detailed. However, their plight is one that has moved many writers, including judges and compilers of official reports, to angry, emotional language. For example:

Hundreds of them are dumb, simple persons, caught in the web of law, unable to comprehend what has happened, what the charge against them is or why they have been sent to jail.

(National Police Commission 1981)

Justice Bhagwati's leading opinion burns with red-hot anger; the Court is appalled and ashamed that such a thing should happen

*Table 2.1*  Selected characteristics of convicted persons in
Indian prisons on 31 December 1980

| Age | No. | % |
|---|---|---|
| Under 16 | 574 | 0.9 |
| 16–20 | 4,845 | 7.6 |
| 21–30 | 21,583 | 33.9 |
| 31–40 | 21,361 | 33.5 |
| 41 and above | 15,336 | 24.1 |
| Total | 63,699 | 100 |
| *Length of sentence* | No. | % |
| Up to and inc. 1 year | 22,915 | 35.8 |
| Over 1–5 years | 9,964 | 15.5 |
| Over 5–10 years | 5,197 | 8.1 |
| Over 10 years | 26,014 | 40.6 |
| Total | 64,090 | 100 |
| *Type of offence* | No. | % |
| Murder/culpable homicide | 29,117 | 45.4 |
| Rape | 811 | 1.2 |
| Dacoity/robbery | 6,005 | 9.4 |
| Burglary/theft | 13,693 | 21.4 |
| Breach of trust/counterfeiting/cheating | 1,134 | 1.8 |
| Prohibition/Gambling/Opium Acts | 3,078 | 4.8 |
| Customs/Excise Acts | 1,558 | 2.4 |
| Prevention of Corruption Act | 217 | 0.3 |
| Indian Railways Act | 2,843 | 4.4 |
| Other | 5,634 | 8.8 |
| Total | 64,090 | 100 |

*Sources:* Adapted from Report of All-Indian Committee on Jail Reform 1980–3 and
Chadha 1983: Appendices

in a democratic, socialist India, over a quarter of a century after
the inception of its Constitution. Such judicial expression of
anger is not to be found anywhere in India, and, one would even
say, the common law world.

(Baxi 1982: 230, describing the *Hussainara* case)

At the end of December 1980, the returns to the Committee on Jail
Reform indicated that almost 7,000 (8 per cent) of the 92,000
undertrials had been in gaol for over one year, and 2,500 of these

had been held for more than two years. The situation was particularly disturbing in the state of Bihar, which alone accounted for three-quarters of the latter group. Moreover, Bihar had been forced a year earlier to release over 27,000 undertrials, following orders from the Supreme Court in *Hussainara* (Shourie 1980: 137–8). The hearing revealed that undertrials had been held in Bihar gaols for up to ten years, in some cases spending years longer on remand than the maximum possible sentence. Justice Bhagwati commented:

> For example, one Lambodar Gorain has been held in Ranchi Jail since 18th June 1970, for an offence under Section 25 of the Arms Act . . . with the result that he has been in prison for eight and a half years for an offence for which even if convicted, he could not have been awarded more than two years imprisonment. . . . What faith would these people have in our system of administration of justice?
>
> (Supreme Court: *H. Khatoon* v. *Home Secretary* SCC 1980(1))

It should be noted that there is a legal limit of ninety days, which can be extended only in exceptional circumstances, for suspects to be remanded in judicial custody pending police investigations and the presentation of a charge-sheet. However, despite this law and despite the publicity following the *Hussainara* case, many magistrates continue to authorize long extensions at the request of the police. Consequently, a large proportion, perhaps the majority, of undertrials have yet to be charged.

There is not space here to delve deeper into the reasons for the unusual profile of the Indian prison population as described above. However, most informed commentators agree that the key factors include the inefficiency, and sometimes corruption, of an outmoded police force, in combination with the failures of a court system clogged up with cases and handicapped by immensely complex procedures.[7] Not only are victims, particularly of personal theft or burglary, usually reluctant to become entangled with the bureaucratic nightmare that can follow the reporting of a crime to the police, but it is extremely difficult to convict anyone who possesses either a good lawyer or 'influence'.[8] Many cases are mysteriously dropped, the vast majority of accused persons, in all but the most minor cases, plead not guilty, and the majority are found not guilty. Broadly speaking, the only people likely to become convicts are the very poor: either sentenced summarily in magistrates' courts for minor offences, or, after long delays, convicted of serious crimes. The undertrial population, too, mainly consists of the most disadvantaged sections of society, who cannot pay the sureties demanded for bail. The more resourceful tend to escape charges through influence over the police, to escape custodial remand through bail, and to escape conviction through employing good lawyers.

Before discussing prison conditions in more depth, an important preliminary point must be considered. It should not be forgotten that although India has made remarkable economic progress over the last thirty years, it is still a Third World country in which enormous numbers of people live in conditions of severe poverty. This means first of all that prisons compete with other government responsibilities for extremely precious resources and secondly that the question of 'less-eligibility' inevitably raises its head. Can prison diets and living conditions reasonably be judged by the same criteria as those in western countries, when the quality of life for the 'honest poor' outside is so much lower? The realistic answer must be 'no', although this does not defeat the argument of Richardson (1985) among others, that the drastic loss of civic rights suffered by prisoners puts a duty upon the state to compensate by giving them 'special rights' when incarcerated. In other words, the less-eligibility argument should never be used to justify deliberate neglect or harsh treatment of prisoners. Thus, for example, while many inmates may sleep in worse conditions outside, this is no argument for making them sleep on concrete if it is not excessively expensive to provide them with cots or hammocks.

Even when making full allowance for the cultural context and resource limitations, nearly all independent commentators agree that, at least until very recently, conditions in Indian prisons have been appalling. The 1983 report of the All-India Committee on Jail Reforms, headed by Justice A.N. Mulla, makes this clear. Every chapter of this carefully researched document, itself a tribute to the democratic institutions and traditions which make India so special among developing countries, reveals further horrors of a harsh and neglected prison system. A few sentences from chapter III, headed 'Realities in Indian Prisons', will give the flavour of the report:

Conditions of living in most of the prisons are sub-human. . . . Shortage of water supply, open drainage systems, conservancy latrines and dearth of scavengers make prison environs unbearable in a large number of institutions . . .

While the lot of the average prisoner leaves much to be desired, that of the criminal lunatic is much worse. These individuals are huddled together under the most unhygienic conditions, totally uncared for and quite frequently ill-treated . . .

Prison industries and work programmes . . . are ill-planned, antiquated, wasteful and unproductive and are little suited to equip inmates with any useful skill . . .

The prison staff has generally become callous and insensitive. It even uses bad characters, hardened criminals and 'dadas' in perpetrating atrocities on other prisoners and indulging in corrupt practices . . .

In most of the prisons, corruption has become a way of life and inmates believe that without taking recourse to corrupt practices they cannot cope with the culture that prevails.

Prisons are run on archaic methods of management. . . . Training of prison personnel has remained woefully neglected . . .

But for making certain general platitudinous statements, [senior prison administrators] could not make any significant contribution in suggesting solutions to the chronic problems of prison management. This is indicative of a very casual and superficial approach to problems of prison at the level of policy formulation in most of the States and Union Territories . . .

After an overall view of the existing conditions in prisons, we are constrained to record that prison organisation in India does not conform to the required standards of a correctional department.

(All-India Committee 1983: paras 3.18–3.45)

Although the most comprehensive, this was only the latest in a long series of hard-hitting reports on Indian prisons, most of which echoed familiar themes. Official recognition of the need for gaol reform dates back to 1919, when a major report by the Indian Jails Committee heralded a change in government pronouncements about the aims of imprisonment, renouncing the retributive philosophy which had been enshrined in policy and legislation since the report of Lord Macauley's Prison Disciplinary Committee in 1838. Macauley's report had rejected reform, education and moral teaching, in favour of a punitive regime based upon deliberately 'dull, monotonous, wearisome and uninteresting tasks'. This had set the tone later reflected in the harsh rules of the Indian Penal Code 1860 (prescribing long sentences of 'rigorous imprisonment'), in the Prisons Act 1894, in gaol manuals allowing cruel punishments for the smallest breach of discipline, and in a lasting policy of spending as little as possible on the gaols. The 1919 report introduced an era of lip-service to 'reform and rehabilitation', but neither the British, preoccupied with 'law and order' as the independence movement gained strength, nor any Indian government after 1947, found the time or the resolve necessary for dismantling the old Draconian system. Even today, most convicts are sentenced to 'rigorous' imprisonment,[9] and, although some revisions are currently being made, the gaols in most states are run according to manuals dating from the nineteenth century.

Critics of Indian prisons have continued for years to point out the incongruity of attempting to run an avowedly 'correctional' prison system with structures, rules and physical conditions created for quite different purposes. Among the most frequently condemned aspects have been the following:

1 Unsuitable buildings, half of them now over fifty years old and 18 per cent over a hundred years;
2 Poor water supply, sanitation, drainage and electrical supply. In 1979, only 15 per cent of gaols had tap water, 33 per cent had septic latrines and 25 per cent were electrified. (However, these are areas currently being improved with central government grants – see below);
3 Poorly funded and poorly organized state management and administration, often in neglected branches of larger departments, employing ignorant, inefficient, and sometimes corrupt staff. Inspector-Generals of Prisons drafted in from other fields with little knowledge of, or interest in, prisons, while 'high flying' young administrators see the prison department as one to be avoided (Sharma 1985);
4 Virtually untrained and sometimes brutal warders, without the influence of a fully-trained national 'cadre' of officers (as in the police) to encourage higher standards and to disseminate new ideas. Assisted often by 'convict warders', who add to an atmosphere of fear and connive in the corruption which is endemic in many institutions. Occasional allegations of torture;

5 Indiscriminate mixing of prisoners of all kinds, with only rudimentary classification, often in overcrowded conditions;
6 Lack of rewarding work, meaningful education, vocational training, 'prison career' planning, or any serious rehabilitative programmes, including provisions for after-care;
7 Poor quality and monotonous diet;
8 Primitive medical facilities and dearth of welfare workers, counsellors or psychiatrists, even where considerable numbers of mentally ill prisoners are held;
9 Capricious and ungenerous systems of furlough, parole and remission;
10 Harsh disciplinary systems giving prisoners few rights of defence, combined with ineffective and unused grievance procedures;
11 Infrequency of inspection, by experts or by appointed visitors, helping to foster a hostile, secretive attitude towards outsiders.

Of course, by no means every one of these problems is to be found in every one of India's hundreds of gaols in its thirty-one independently governed states. While some are grossly overcrowded, others are half-empty; some are riddled with corruption but others are tightly run; and while some are undoubtedly filthy and unhealthy in the extreme, others are kept very clean. The gaol I visited was neither overcrowded nor filthy. But although I chose it virtually at random, this does not make it 'typical', any more than the horrific Bihar gaol described by Sinha (1978) in which 143 people had died within three years.[10] In the face of such variety, it may appear that any attempt to generalize from a description of one institution is doomed to failure. Nevertheless, certain features of the gaol I saw seemed to reveal something more fundamental about imprisonment than did the state of the drains or other physical conditions, which may vary widely between institutions or, indeed, in the same institution over time. I was particularly struck by aspects of the regime that, to some Indian colleagues with whom I discussed them, were 'routine', but to a foreigner seemed to reveal fundamental assumptions in the country about how prisoners should be treated. The following account summarizes the factual information I obtained about the prison, as well as the general impressions I gained during the necessarily short time I was able to spend inside it.

## II CONDITIONS IN A CENTRAL GAOL

Few visitors are welcome in Indian prisons, and it is particularly difficult for foreigners to achieve access. I was fortunate enough, with the help of contacts in the academic world, to persuade the relevant central government and state authorities to allow me to visit an institution informally, on condition that neither the prison nor any individual would be identified in anything I wrote. In the end, I spent two afternoons in a central gaol (the highest category of prison, intended primarily for long-termers) in a major town in the south of India. The first afternoon was spent mainly with the Superintendent and the second incorporated a full and relatively leisurely tour of the prison, seeing whatever I wished. Naturally, such visits can allow only the most superficial understanding of prison life, any conversations with prisoners and warders being cursory and inhibited by the presence of a senior officer. Nevertheless, the staff were open and co-operative and I found the visit productive, gleaning more information and obtaining clearer impressions than I originally expected. Inevitably, I saw the prison through the eyes of a western visitor, but after three months in India I had acquired at least a superficial understanding of the country and its penal philosophy.

The gaol was situated not far from the centre of a large and fast-growing industrial town. Built around the turn of the century, it had been designed originally as a soldiers' barracks. There was an outer compound, in which relatives waited for their turn to speak to prisoners through the bars of the main prison. The gate to this compound was guarded by an unfriendly warder in khaki uniform, similar to that worn by police and soldiers. He refused to let us pass, and my companion and I waited an hour before being rescued by a passing senior officer. While waiting we watched a small number of trusted prisoners in ragged white cotton shirts, shorts and head-dress come and go apparently freely through the outer gate, engaged in errands or in work in the nearby gardens.

The main prison, into which few outsiders were allowed, was guarded by armed officers. It was divided into three compounds, as well as a small section for high security prisoners (there were only three of the latter at the time I visited). One of the compounds held primarily undertrial prisoners, one convicted short-termers, and the third convicted long-termers. However, this was not a strict division, and there was a certain amount of mixing of categories, mainly because of the large numbers of undertrials. The long-termers were housed chiefly in single cells, the others in dormitories containing forty 'beds' (or stone slabs). Most of the buildings in the prison were single-storey.

At the time of my visit, there were about 600 prisoners in the prison: 350 undertrials and 250 convicted prisoners. This was nearly 50 per cent higher than the latest official statistics for the prison that I was able to obtain: on 31 December 1987, just over a year earlier, there had been a population of 405. The official return did not give any details about the population on that, or any other, day, but there was a breakdown of the characteristics of all prisoners admitted during 1987. The year's admissions had consisted of 947 convicts, 2,018 undertrials and 15 detenus. No fewer than 708 of the convicts (75 per cent) had been aged 31 or over, and 573 (61 per cent) had been illiterate. As one would expect, the majority of the sentenced prisoners coming in through the gates had received short terms, but 121 (13 per cent) had been admitted to serve sentences over five years and 84 of these had received life imprisonment for murder. Only 23 were classified as 'habitual offenders' by dint of having one or more previous convictions of substance.

To guard the 600 prisoners, there were just under 200 uniformed warders, who worked three eight-hour shifts. They were not required to escort prisoners from court or to other prisons, this being a police responsibility in India, so during the day there might be 70 or so warders in the prison at any one time.

We went first to the short-termers' section, which consisted of several barracks in a surprisingly spacious compound. Nearly all prisoners were out of their cells, either employed in the workshops (see later) or standing around talking or exercising on the sparsely grassed areas between the barracks. Despite this apparent freedom, the discipline was clearly strict. There were numerous warders in sight, all armed with sticks, and every prisoner within range stood to attention and saluted as the Deputy Superintendent passed.

The barracks were single-storey huts, each with forty raised stone slabs to serve as beds. Prisoners were allowed no personal possessions such as photographs of their families, let alone items like radios or hobby materials, so, apart from some religious paintings on the walls, the dormitories had an austere look, each 'bed' furnished only with a jute mat and pillow, together with the prisoner's plate, spoon and mug. At the end of each barracks were latrines, which, like all in the prison, drained into septic tanks. The latrines were generally clean.

The other two sections of the prison also contained barracks, but many of the long-term prisoners lived in blocks of single cells. These were quite large, and some prisoners chose to share with two others rather than face solitude. The cells were generally bare with stone 'beds', but were clean and had integral toilets and water taps.

The prison kitchen was located in the short-termers' compound. Later in the afternoon I saw a meal for all 600 prisoners being cooked in one gigantic iron pot over a blazing fire. The pot was taller than a man, and a prisoner had to climb up on a table in order to extract a sample with a huge ladle. It looked and tasted exactly the same as the previous day's meal which I had sampled in the Superintendent's office – a medium-hot vegetable curry containing a mixture of root and leafy vegetables. There was also a bitter tamarind soup. A group of prisoners was carefully picking foreign bodies from a mound of rice before cooking.

The diet in this, as in all Indian prisons, was laid down in very precise terms. The entitlements per prisoner were printed in English and in the local language on a large notice outside the kitchen. The following was the diet laid down for working prisoners (those not working received 100 grams less rice per day):

| ITEMS | QUANTITY IN GRAMS |
|---|---|
| (Per head per day) | |
| Rice or wheat | 700 |
| Dall (not to be issued on Sundays) | 100 |
| Vegetables | 250 |
| Groundnut oil or any other substitute | 30 |
| Tamarind | 20 |
| Fuel (firewood or any other substitute) | 700 |
| Salt | 35 |
| Mutton with bones or any other non-vegetarian dish (weekly once) | 175 |
| Onions (to be issued on Sundays) | 15 |
| Chillies | 10 |
| Turmeric | 2 |
| Garlic | 4 |

| Coriander | 4 |
| Chillies to be issued on Sundays | |
| (extra besides the quantity of 10 grams) | 5 |
| Milk (to be converted into buttermilk | |
| or curd) | 70 ml. |

On Sundays and on nine festival days each year, prisoners received a special diet, including 175 grams of meat per man. For the festivals, there was a budget allocation of one rupee per head (about 4p in UK currency). In order to gain some idea of the adequacy of the diet, I asked several people from poor families outside how much rice they ate and whether they would find the prison food acceptable. It appeared that, in terms of weight, it was roughly the equivalent of an agricultural labourer's daily intake of rice. It was also over 50 per cent more than that laid down in codes for the relief of famine as a basic subsistence diet (Kynch 1989). The main criticisms made by most people I spoke to who had experience of prison food concerned not its quantity but its quality. The food was described as tasteless and monotonous, and often cold by the time it reached people housed some distance from the kitchens. More important, it was not high in protein or calories, and many of the longer-term prisoners looked thin and weak. Of course, it might be argued that most of them come from very poor rural areas, and that their diets outside would be equally poor, if not poorer, in nutritional value. But these 'less-eligibility' arguments are surely at their weakest when applied to food, and virtually untenable when one is talking about people incarcerated for fourteen years or more.

It should be noted that, while the budgets and weight of food items were calculated per prisoner, this did not mean that each inmate was given an individually weighed portion: the uncooked food was simply weighed in bulk on leaving the stores for the kitchen. I am unaware of any allegations of malpractice at the prison I visited, but it has often been claimed elsewhere that frauds are common among both staff and prisoners responsible for storing, weighing and distributing food, and that the actual consumption per prisoner can be up to 20 per cent below that laid down in the regulations. To these risks of malpractice can be added further risks in discrimination further down the line. Inmates were divided into groups of five, and usually lived, worked and ate as a group. The leader of each group collected the food and was responsible for distributing it among his 'team'. Obviously, this kind of system allows opportunities for abuses and oppression of some prisoners by others.

The practice of giving some inmates power over others is not unusual in Indian prisons. As elsewhere, the gaol I visited appointed 'convict overseers' to assist the staff, a system much criticized in recent years. However, there were only four of these, and their role was restricted to supervising prisoners in work and vocational activities, rather than the disciplinary roles undertaken by the more controversial 'convict warders' employed in many other gaols. Although they had no power to punish prisoners themselves, the overseers reported any misdemeanours to staff and their word would almost always be taken against that of another prisoner. They therefore had a certain amount of power over others and were also known to receive 'perks', for example extra food from the kitchen. A healthier kind of 'prisoner power' was to be found in the 'panchayat' system, whereby prisoners elected representatives to put their collective views to the Superintendent. Elections for six places on the panchayat were held every six months, staff reserving the right to exclude from consideration any prisoner they considered unsuitable.

## III  WORK, EDUCATION, WELFARE, PAROLE

The normal daily routine for a convicted prisoner was constructed as follows:

| | |
|---|---|
| 05.30–07.00 | Reveille, ablutions, breakfast |
| 07.00–11.00 | Work |
| 11.00–13.00 | Lunch and rest |
| 13.00–16.30 | Work |
| 16.30–17.30 | Recreation |
| 17.30–18.30 | Evening meal |
| 18.30–21.30 | Locked in cells/barracks, lights on |
| 21.30 | Lights out |

All convicted prisoners sentenced to rigorous imprisonment (the great majority) were obliged to work seven-and-a-half hours per day. Undertrials and any short-termers sentenced to simple imprisonment were allocated only domestic duties. They could, however, volunteer for work, which entitled them to wages and to a better diet (the same as convicted prisoners).

There were five main types of 'vocational' work in the prison: weaving, carpentry, printing, bookbinding and textile work. However, not all of these were 'going concerns' at any particular time. At the end of 1987, the distribution of jobs among convicts was recorded as follows:

*Maintenance*

| | |
|---|---|
| Convict overseers | 4 |
| Cleaners, sweepers | 39 |
| Repairs | 1 |
| Cooks | 8 |
| Other | 19 |

*Vocational*

| | |
|---|---|
| Agriculture/gardening | 15 |
| Weaving | 23 |
| Tailoring | 2 |
| Blacksmithy | 1 |
| Carpentry | 39 |
| Printing/bookbinding | 1 |
| Oil expelling | 2 |
| Jute work | 14 |
| *Total* | 168 |

Normally, the 'vocational' jobs, which carried slightly higher wages, were given only to men serving over two years, and the Superintendent stated that little attempt was made to 'rehabilitate' those sentenced to less. The equipment in all the workshops was rudimentary, but items of reasonable quality were produced and sold, some of them on a stall outside the front gate of the prison. In most cases, prisoners worked in their groups of five, and were paid (or not) according to how well the group performed. In the weaving shop, for example, prisoners were paid three rupees each day, but only if the group completed thirty yards of woven sheeting. Staff estimated that this very stiff target was attained relatively rarely, so that, at most, one in five of the prisoners actually received pay on any one day. When they did enough to earn wages, they were allowed to keep or spend half, the other half being saved for them on their release. The level of pay, which fell from three to two rupees per day for non-vocational work, can be judged from a comparison of the prison wage with the typical wage of an agricultural labourer in the area. The latter would receive around fourteen rupees per day.

The allocation of work was in some cases based upon people's skills outside; for example, prisoners who had been barbers, washermen, gardeners or 'sweepers' (refuse collectors and cleaners from the lower castes) were given similar jobs if available, but, generally speaking, new inmates were assigned a task without much deliberation or consultation. Thereafter, it was difficult for them to change. As the Superintendent put it, 'Rehabilitation means learning to work', which included work which they did not like or to which they were not suited. This reflects a common tendency in India to think of rigorous imprisonment and vocational work as meaning the same thing: little distinction is made between punishment and rehabilitation in the prison context.

There was one teacher employed in the prison, who undertook education at all levels from basic literacy to assisting with open university degrees. He also distributed library books to those who asked for them – although I saw few books in the cells or barracks and it was stated that few prisoners were interested in reading. Prisoners were not normally allowed to visit the library to choose their own books. But although the educational services were supplied to only a few inmates, several of these were undertaking advanced work: three had completed BAs over the past few years, another an MA, and nine were embarking upon university degrees by correspondence.

Welfare provision, apart from that provided by the prison staff themselves, was non-existent. There were two posts allocated for social workers, but these had not been filled for a long time. The only recourse for prisoners with social or practical problems, including those involving families outside, was to make an application to see the Superintendent or another senior officer. There was a prison hospital with twelve beds, but this had little equipment and only basic drugs. Seriously ill prisoners were transferred to outside hospitals. In 1987, 233 had been admitted at some time into the prison hospital.

The main recreational activities in the prison were volley-ball, ring tennis, chess, kabaddi and other board games, but limited numbers of prisoners actually engaged in them. There was also an outdoor stage on which occasional concerts, plays, or other entertainment or religious functions were held.

There are in India a variety of systems of home leave, furlough, early release and parole, but in practice relatively few prisoners benefit. During 1987–8 in the prison I visited, twenty-three prisoners had been granted home leave, mainly for reasons of death or serious illness in their families. Early release was possible on the recommendation of an Advisory Board, made up of representatives from various agencies, but in 1987, while 458 were released on expiry of their sentence, none at all appeared to have been granted early release on licence. (Similarly, Datir (1978: 245) found that only five of 644 released prisoners in a sample in Maharastra had been granted this.) Most, however, had earned remission, which is given at a rate of five days per month, so long as the prisoner works to a satisfactory standard. Lifers were entitled after two years to apply for furlough to maintain contact with their families, but this was in the hands of the police department, not the prison authorities, and was rarely granted – a matter of some concern to the gaol Superintendent.

Finally, formal punishments were used relatively rarely. During 1987, only twenty-six prisoners had been officially punished, twenty-five of these for 'minor' offences – although these included fighting, stealing and 'sodomy'. The punishments included forfeiture of remission, single cell confinements, restrictions upon access to the canteen and, more controversially, the stopping of letters and visits for up to a month. (In normal circumstances each prisoner was allowed one visit and one letter per week.) On rare occasions, too, handcuffs could be applied as a punishment. The rarity of formal disciplinary hearings is perhaps one indication of the strict control of inmates achieved by the continual presence of considerable numbers of warders armed with long sticks. It may also reflect the nature of the inmate population. As one informant put it, most are not 'hardened criminals' but uneducated rural dwellers who would rarely show open disrespect to people of higher caste or to those they perceive as 'sahibs'.

One must, of course, be cautious in drawing conclusions from only two visits to an institution, but I can perhaps summarize my general impressions. The basic living conditions were clearly above average for Indian prisons, judging from published and oral accounts of those elsewhere. In terms of space, sanitation and general cleanliness, conditions seemed acceptable, and I have certainly seen worse in British prisons. The food, although mainly low in nutritive value, unappetizing and depressingly monotonous, was at least adequate in quantity. On the other hand, the features which stood out most starkly to a western visitor were the harshness of the regime, the lack of stimulation for long-term prisoners, the absence of welfare provisions, and the exclusion of even minor personal comforts such as the display of family mementos and the pursuit of cell hobbies.

Although some lip-service is now being paid to the concept of rehabilitation within prisons, there was little evidence of serious efforts to prepare prisoners for life outside. The lack of welfare officers, the rarity of home leave, the concept of visits and letter-writing as a privilege which could be withdrawn as a punishment, and the denial of permission to keep family photographs, were all indications of an absence of serious interest in helping to maintain a prisoner's contacts with the outside world. Similarly, 'vocational' training was regarded more as a means of making prisoners work hard than of training them for a task to which they were individually suited. And the absence of systematic programmes to teach basic literacy added to the impression that the prison was regarded in reality as little more than a 'warehouse' for inmates, not a vehicle for their improvement. Above all, there seemed to be little recognition of the special needs of people who were destined to spend very long periods behind bars: the long-termers were treated not very differently from the short-termers, and relatively little thought seemed to have been given to the risk of mental deterioration in an environment without stimulus. Thus, while the basic living conditions were markedly better than I had expected, it has to be recorded that the 'psychological' character of the institution (as, I suspect, in most prisons in India) appeared to me harsh, negative and even cruel.

## IV PROSPECTS FOR REFORM

While the institution I visited may not have been entirely 'typical' – indeed, was in a state with a relatively good record on prisons – the above observations highlight some of the difficult issues facing penal reformers in India. Prisons not only carry the weight of a bleak, punitive tradition dating from the days of the British, but the long years of neglect and lack of investment mean that any significant reforms demand a massive injection of resources. The fundamental problem here is that, as in many other countries, prison reform occupies one of the lowest rungs on the ladder of political priorities. India's major government policy is set and its large-scale capital expenditure is committed in a series of Five Year Plans. Unsurprisingly, these are dominated by schemes for economic development. Prisons, being regarded by most planners and politicians as 'non-productive' (short-sighted a view as this may be), did not until very recently achieve even token inclusion in a Five Year Plan, and this came only after a lengthy battle by individuals within the Ministries of Home Affairs and Welfare to include a meaningful package for development in the correctional field. Budgets for prisons have hardly kept pace with inflation, and, despite occasional lip-service commitment to reform, the policy of the British before 1947 – to run gaols as cheaply as possible – has not changed significantly in practice (Baxi 1982; Khan and Chilad 1982; Bhatacharya 1985; Gokhale and Sohoni 1988).

The problem was exacerbated by the decision in 1950 to leave prisons as primarily the province of the states, which gives the central government something of an excuse for its half-hearted approach to reform. A further deep-seated reason for neglect lies in the unforgiving attitudes of the general population towards criminals, which, although fostered and maintained by the British, existed long before and after they left (cf. Chhrabra 1970). Many prisoners continue to be rejected by their local community upon release, there is very little voluntary involvement in after-care, and, except when political activists are imprisoned, few public pressure groups demand reform.

Criminologists, too, have largely neglected the prisons. In an excellent review of the literature, Srivastava (1982) concluded that, while there were some useful Ph.D. theses, only two published books (her own (1977) and that of Singh (1978)) were based substantially upon primary empirical research within prisons. The vast majority of academic writers, as I discovered myself in a trawl of more recent literature, tend to recycle old material, relying upon out-of-date statistics and official reports. This has greatly reduced their potential for instigating change. Instead, the only effective exposure of prison conditions and pressure for reform have come from journalists, lawyers, judges and, indeed, international organizations such as Amnesty International. For example, ex-detenus such as Nayar (1978), Tyler (1977) and Kumar (1979) have written graphic accounts of their time in gaol, another journalist Sheela Barse has fought determinedly (including initiating law-suits) for the removal of children from gaols, and Justices Bhagwati and Krishna Iyer made wide-ranging pronouncements – as well as damning general comments – in celebrated Supreme Court cases such as *Hussainara Khatoon* and *Sunil Batra*.[11]

Despite these praiseworthy efforts, only the tip of the iceberg has been noticeably affected. The hugely daunting size of the problem – nearly 1,200 gaols under the control of thirty-one different states – ensures that even unequivocal instructions from the Supreme Court are anything but universally implemented. Unless there are local people with the time, resources and energy to file petitions of contempt, matters are likely to remain unchanged in many parts of the country (Dhagamwar 1987).[12]

The one glimmer of light on the horizon at present is the possibility of a positive reaction by the government to the Mulla Committee's comprehensive report. Certain periods in the past have seen minor bursts of prison reform, and it may be that this will produce another. One such followed the 1919 Indian Jails Committee report, and another came shortly after Independence; many of the new leaders had spent time in gaols, and devoted some attention to the problem in the 1950s (including the drawing up of a Model Prison Manual in 1959). The flurry of critical publications by ex-detenus after the Emergency helped to attract some extra finance towards prisons, as well as fuelling the pressure which led to the setting up of Justice Mulla's committee. Khan and Chilad (1982: 49) saw these developments as the 'modest beginning' of a new phase in prison reform, in which, at last, 'institutional correction was accorded the status of an *issue*, worthy of being discussed by the political executive and the bureaucracy'.

In the six years since the Mulla Committee's report, there has been a certain amount of further progress, including increases in the prison budget, some new instructions from the central government to the states, and the setting up of a small policy section within the Ministry of Home Affairs to consider the implementation of the recommendations. The Eighth Finance Commission in 1985[13] recommended the allocation of more funds for the restructuring of prison buildings, and the Ministry of Welfare put forward a plan for improving the welfare of prisoners, including some attention to after-care, under the Seventh Five Year Plan. Instructions to the states included a timetable for the rewriting of outdated gaol manuals and recommendations for the improvement of staff training, as well as a demand for quarterly reports on progress.

It is not yet clear whether this is the beginning of significant changes, or merely another short-lived period of interest. It has to be noted that gaol conditions are no longer newsworthy and the clamour for reform has largely faded. After six years, the Mulla report is still 'under consideration' by the state governments, and has yet to be laid before Parliament. Despite the encouraging signs mentioned earlier, there is a danger that it may meet a similar fate to all its worthy predecessors.

In sum, effective penal reform will not be achieved until the central government takes it really seriously and

1  Injects a vastly increased amount of money into the prison system;[14]
2  Enacts major new legislation, completely recasting the punitive Indian Penal Code 1860 and Prison Act 1894;
3  Creates a national cadre of properly trained prison officers;
4  Sets up effective inspection machinery.

Ultimately, this may be best achieved by transferring full responsibility for prisons from the states to the central government, or, if this remains politically unfeasible, by building more federal prisons as 'models' for the remainder (an engine of reform in other countries with a similar federal structure).

Such a programme of reform requires a firm 'political will', which in turn depends upon demands from the people. Unfortunately, in present-day India, despite its openness in many areas of government and its generally good record on human rights, the state of the prisons remains a rather shameful secret, surfacing now and then, but basically an issue in which neither the politicians, nor the vocal pressure groups, nor the public, have an abiding interest or concern.

## NOTES

1  For example, the National Security Act and the Conservation of Foreign Exchange and the Prevention of Smuggling Activities Act.
2  This occurred most dramatically during the 'Emergency' of 1975–7, when thousands of the government's political opponents, including academics and journalists, were arrested and detained. More recently,

both Amnesty International and the US State Department have accused India of violating human rights, particularly in regard to suppression of terrorism in the Punjab.

3 The traditional name for gangs of violent robbers. 'Dacoity' is an offence under the Indian penal code.

4 The terms are used in the Indian Lunacy Act 1912, which has not been revised.

5 'Children' are defined in the Indian penal system as boys under the age of 16 and girls under 18.

6 'Sub-gaols', some of which are very small, make up over two-thirds of all gaols in India. Many are managed by part-time superintendents, and some are, in effect, run by the local police (Baxi 1982: 178–83).

7 Gokhale and Sohoni (1988: 170) note that in 1974, the cases of 72 per cent of the total persons arrested remained 'pending' at the end of that year.

8 It is by no means uncommon in criminal cases, including murder, in which local politics are involved (and many assaults in India are connected with politically-motivated disputes) or in which people with local influence are involved, for pressure to be put upon senior police officers to drop the charges. If this pressure comes from senior enough level, particularly in the governing party, it is very difficult to resist (see, for example, Sharma 1977; National Police Commission 1981; Baxi 1982; Gupta 1988). It is also widely believed that the more professional thieves 'pay off' the police to escape arrest.

9 Convicted persons in India are sentenced either to rigorous or to simple imprisonment, the latter reserved mainly for minor offenders, who are not required to work. Of the convicted population at any one time, no more than 6–7 per cent will be serving simple imprisonment.

10 Baxi writes: 'One would like to believe that Seraikela jail does not represent the typical Indian prison. Unfortunately, all available evidence (random and sketchy though it is, of necessity) reminds us that India is a sub-continent full of Seraikelas'. However, this is not a fair conclusion from the other evidence he presents. Nor does it fit, for example, with Datir's evidence (1978: 378) of a low death rate in Maharastra prisons (32 deaths in 1970 out of an average daily population of 14,809).

11 The *H. Khatoon* case (see earlier) resulted in the release of thousands of undertrials, and *Sunil Batra* (All India Report 1978 Sc. 1675 and 1980 Sc. 1579) outlawed the indiscriminate use of solitary confinement and bars and fetters.

12 Dhagamwar (1987) writes: 'Justice Bhagwati's fond hopes of the High Courts were to be disappointed. As the months passed the unpleasant truth began to emerge. The Supreme Court was unable to discipline the executive.' Similar problems in the implementation of court decisions have been met in the field of prison reform in the USA. There, courts have sometimes appointed 'masters' to oversee the implementation of their decisions (Bronstein and Morgan 1985).

13 In 1978, the Seventh Finance Commission had intervened in the prisons area for the first time, recommending an allocation of Rs. 480 million (about £20 million sterling) by the central government to states with serious deficiencies in water supply, electricity and sanitation in their prisons, as well as for new building.

14 A good illustration of governmental approach is the conference of Chief Secretaries of the states in 1979, which was the first time 'the top bureaucracy in a country came round a table to discuss a relatively insignificant subject like jails' (Khan and Chilad 1982: 48). While agreeing upon reforms, including the adoption of the Model Prison Manual, they failed to seek the necessary additional funds.

## REFERENCES

All-India Committee on Jail Reforms (1983) *Report of All-India Committee on Jail Reforms 1980–3* (Justice A.N. Mulla, Chairman), New Delhi: Government of India.

Baxi, U. (1982) *The Crisis of the Indian Legal System*, Delhi: Bikas Publishing House.

Bhatacharya, S.K. (1985) 'An assessment of the institutional treatment programmes for adults and juveniles', *Indian Journal of Criminology and Criminalistics* 3, 4, pp. 136–41.

Bronstein, A. and Morgan, R. (1985) 'Prisoners and the courts: the United States experience', in M. Maguire, J. Vagg and R. Morgan (eds) *Accountability and Prisons*, London: Tavistock.

Chadha, K. (1983) *The Indian Jail*, Delhi: Vikas.

Chhrabra, K.S. (1970) *Quantum of Punishment in Criminal Law in India*, Chandigarh: Punjab University Publication Bureau.

*Crime in India 1983* (1988), New Delhi: Government of India.

Datir, R.N. (1978) *Prison as a Social System*, Bombay: Popular Press.

Dhagamwar, V. (1987) 'The disadvantaged and the law', paper to workshop *Poverty in India: Research and Policy*, Queen Elizabeth House, Oxford, 1–6 October 1987.

Diaz (1977) 'The forgotten man of the criminal justice system', *Journal of Correctional Work*.

Gokhale, S.D. and Sohoni, N.K. (1988) 'Whither correction?', in S.V. Rao (ed.) *Perspectives in Criminology*, New Delhi: Vikas.

Gupta, A.S. (1988) 'Law and order in a democratic society', in S.V. Rao (ed.) *Perspectives in Criminology*, New Delhi: Vikas.

Khan, M.Z. and Chilad, B.S. (1982) 'Policy shifts in institutional correction in India', *Indian Journal of Social Work* 43, no. 1, pp. 39–51.

Krishna, Iyer, Justice V.R. (1988) 'From Macauley to Mahatma: an Indian criminological odyssey', *Indian Journal of Criminology* 16, no. 2.

Kumar, S. (1979) *A Chief Minister's Prison Diary*, Delhi: Vikas.

Kynch, J. (1989) 'Scarcities, distress and crime in British India', paper to 7th World Congress on Rural Sociology, Bologna, July 1988.

National Police Commission (1981) *Compendium of Observations and Recommendations of the National Police Commission*, New Delhi: Government of India.

Nayar, K. (1978) *In Jail*, New Delhi: Vikas.

Reckless, W.D. (1952) *Report on Jail Administration in India*, Delhi: Government Publication Division.

Richardson, G. (1985) 'The case for prisoners' rights', in M. Maguire, J. Vagg and R. Morgan (eds) *Accountability and Prisons*, London: Tavistock.

Sharma, P.D. (1977) *Indian Police: A Development Approach*, New Delhi: Uppal.

Sharma, P.D. (1985) *Police and Criminal Justice Administration in India*, New Delhi: Uppal.

Shourie, A. (1980) *Institutions under the Janata Rule*, New Delhi.

Shukla, K.S. (1980) in T.N. Chaturvedi and S.K. Chandra (eds) 'Correctional administration in India – research trends and priorities', in *Social Administration: Direction and Change*, New Delhi: Indian Institute of Public Administration.

Shukla, K.S. (ed.) (1987) *The Other Side of Development: Social and Psychological Implications*, New Delhi: Sage.

Sinha, S. (1978) 'The horrors of Seraikela Jail', *Economic and Political Weekly* 13: 1,165.

Singh, I.J. (1978) *Indian Prison: A Sociological Enquiry*, Delhi: Concept Publishing Co.

Srivastava, S.P. (1977) *Indian Prison Community*, Lucknow: Pustak Kendra.

Srivastava, S.P. (1982) 'Research on correctional structures and administration in India', *Indian Journal of Criminology and Criminalistics* 2, no. 2, pp. 119–39.

Trivedi, B.V. (1978) *Prison Administration in India*, New Delhi: Uppal.

Tyler, M. (1977) *My Years in an Indian Prison*, Bombay: B.I. Publications.

# Chapter Three

# THE SLUZEWIEC PRISON IN WARSAW, POLAND

*A penal labour centre, or 'half-open' prison*

MONIKA PLATEK

## INTRODUCTION

A statement that prisons can be found all over the world would be a truism were it not for a certain reflection related to it. Wherever they are, prisons serve the purpose of restricting their inmates' freedom; but the interpretations of the functions and aims officially attributed to them vary according to each state's institutional and legal system. Also, the tasks prisons actually fulfil behind their external, officially specified, aims vary greatly from state to state.

Prisons have certain features in common:

- they do exist in every country;
- they serve as political instruments;
- their officially proclaimed aims are not the only ones they have;
- both the official and the actually fulfilled aims undergo changes that reflect socio-political changes in the societies in which they function;
- in depriving their inmates of liberty they cause a life-threatening and complex affliction.

Thus a description of just one Polish prison will be a picture of a particular reality and an example of prison and imprisonment in Poland. But it will have to leave out the innate socio-political problems of the Polish prison system which deserve a separate and comprehensive discussion, but can only be mentioned here.

In order to achieve a balance, it might be worth while considering the data that characterize the whole of the Polish prison system before we pass the gate leading to the Sluzewiec Prison in Warsaw.

# BASIC INFORMATION ON PRISONS AND PENITENTIARY POLICY IN POLAND

For many years, penal institutions, their population, state of repair, and tasks they fulfilled were a taboo subject in post-war Poland. Some researchers interested in this subject were joined after 1956[1] by a group of students from the Students' Penitentiary Club, which had been founded by an ex-convict who had spent many years in prison during the Stalinist era. They had varying success trying to get inside prisons and to study the prison reality.

It was only in the years 1980–1, in the period of Solidarity, that the size of the prison population was made public for the first time, as well as information about the inmates' living conditions and about the protests that took place in prisons all over Poland in that period. For the first time, too, society itself demanded an improvement in the prisoners' situation. From 1945, the average number of prisoners in Poland has been higher than 100,000. The rate of prisoners per 100,000 of the population was about 300, and after the introduction of the new penal code in 1970 the average prison term exceeded 27 months. In 1981 the number of prisoners went down, but this proved a temporary reduction only. In 1982 the situation was back at 'normal'; the fact that prisons and detention centres were grossly overpopulated was carefully passed over in silence.

The process initiated in the Solidarity period was felt several years later. This time not only society but also the prison system was ripe for reform. Struggling with overpopulation, a shortage of trained staff made worse by more staff resignations, and economic problems, the prisons themselves decided to introduce changes. This process has been encouraged by more open access to previously secret data.

### The prison population in Poland

A report on the state of prisons in Poland, prepared in January 1989 by the Central Prison Management and accepted by the Minister of Justice (to whom prisons have been accountable since 1956), contains the following statement: 'A chronic overpopulation of prison units has been a permanent feature of the system throughout the post-war period. Amnesty acts reduced the populations of detention centres and prisons but for very short periods.'[2] In April 1986, the number of prisoners in Poland went up to 116,000, which made another amnesty act necessary.[3] Passed in July 1986, it reduced the prison population to 102,000. From then on, for the first time in the post-war history of the Polish prison system, the number of prisoners has been going down. This is a result both of changes in penal law, and of a changing sentencing policy. The latter change resulted in a broader use of probation, reduced number of arrests, sentencing of women to prison terms becoming exceptional, and less frequent prison sentences for unintentional offenders, young adults and first offenders. As a result the rate of prisoners per 100,000 of the population is now 177. Hardly a reason to feel satisfied or proud (the world index being calculated at about 100); but in the Polish conditions, this is indeed a positive change.[4]

One should bear it in mind, however, when discussing the prison system that the size of the prison population is only one of the elements in the total picture. Just as essential are data on the prisons' estate and the condition and standard of prison staff.

## The prison estate

According to the data for December 1988, the prison system included 149 basic units: 67 remand prisons and 82 penal institutions for sentenced prisoners; there are also 66 external units under the direct management of prisons and detention centres and 8 'social adjustment centres'; the latter are compulsory for recidivists who have been termed as such by the court, and who spend up to five years there after serving their prison sentence.

About 70 per cent of prisons were built before the First World War, in the 19th or 18th century; some are even older. So, as can be expected, they are in a very bad state of repair. According to the Central Prison Management, nineteen of them are unfit for use (which does not prevent their being just as overcrowded as any other prison).[5] Twenty-six prisons are badly in need of improvement, and in the case of six of them, not even that would help, as they are beyond any repair. Sixteen prisons lack a sewage system, and five lack central heating. All of them are big institutions where 2,000 inmates, on average, have been detained.

A peculiar feature of the Polish, as well as the East-European, prison system is its connection with the state economy. Formally, it follows from the provision of the penal code which speaks of resocialization of prisoners through work. This slogan has been bandied about and the term 'resocialization' abused, until it is void of any meaning in Polish penitentiary practice; the authorities have exploited prisoners, sometimes quite openly, as a cheap or free workforce. It was, and often still is, a thoughtless and wasteful exploitation, one that ruins health, deprives the prisoners of any motivation to work, prejudices them against society, fails to add to their development or, usually, to their qualifications.

The Polish prison system is a big industrial tycoon, owner of 61 self-dependent production units. Of these, 48 are industrial units (26 factories and 22 auxiliary industrial farms); there are also four agricultural and nine building enterprises. All of them together can employ about 26,000 prisoners. A very large group of about 30,000 prisoners work outside prison, building harbours, steelworks and houses, or are employed in mines, ironworks and various factories. There is also a broad category of jobs performed 'quite free' (that is, the state does not pass on the cost) because the work is not concerned directly with 'production'. This group is given the euphemistic name of 'public works'; it includes building roads, laying railway tracks, land reclamation, installation of high-voltage line supports, work at distribution depots. Leaving the details aside, it could be said without exaggeration that the persistence of the very large prison population was due to its existence as an inexhaustible source of labour, to be freely disposed of by the authorities.[6] The crisis of the Polish economy and the resulting need to change production methods and the style of management also helped to make possible the long-demanded prison reform.

That reform is above all manifest in the trend towards reducing the prison population. A provision was introduced in 1986 that was truly revolutionary for the Polish conditions: the living space per prisoner should be at least 2.5 sq.m. The main effect of this during the first eighteen months of its operation was a reduction of the prison population by about half; this was achieved first of all through the use of various forms of release. The population went down to about 60,000. In addition there was a retreat from the assertion, as emphatic as it was preposterous, that a prisoner is treated as a normal employee. The problem has at last been acknowledged of paying prisoners less or not paying them at all just because they are prisoners. Employment in prison is not added to the prisoner's qualifications for entitlement to benefits; consequently, his salary is lower and he has to work longer before he can retire. Prisoners get no money during justified absence. So there is too wide a discrepancy between the apparent meaning of 'resocialization through work' and the term as it works out in practice.

The crisis is such that the prison management itself is now trying to equalize conditions for prisoners and other employees.

### Prison staff in Poland

The changes now introduced in the prison system are also aimed at checking the loss of prison staff. There are about 27,000 regular posts in the prison system, but it has always suffered staff shortages, particularly of well-trained and educated employees. What probably induced some of them to take a job in prison were the higher than average wages and the earlier chance of getting proper housing. This compensated for the disadvantages of service – its low status and unpopularity in society, the need to be on duty for long periods if required, mental fatigue, and so on. Today, however, owing to spiralling inflation, the wages of prison staff are not as attractive as they used to be; the general crisis is also apparent in the prison system's housing shortage and lack of financial means to develop building. An additional burden for the staff is the paramilitary nature of service and the permanent conflict between the educational staff, who amount to about 10 per cent of all prison employees, and the security staff, who are over 50 per cent. Those who quit tend to be aged under 30 and have worked for five years on average. The deteriorating staff situation and unattractive conditions of work intensify the negative attitude of those who stay on.

Thus at the beginning of the 1980s, the prison system was in a situation where changes became both urgent and necessary. The first attempt at solving the crisis by means of increased repression, as used repeatedly in the past, failed this time. The times had changed: Polish society after 1980 was different from society before.[7] But several years passed before those in power who influence the country's penitentiary policy came to understand this.

## THE SLUZEWIEC PRISON IN WARSAW

The above introduction, though short, was needed for a proper appraisal of the processes that are now in progress in the Polish prison system. They will now be illustrated through one penal institution, which differs from other prisons but is not extreme in any way.

Situated on the outskirts of Warsaw, it was built for the prisoners of war who once cleared Warsaw of rubble. Its eight narrow barracks with no sewer system were initially to be used for a short time only, and pulled down afterwards. Instead, in 1951, they were separated from one another by internal walls and tall wire fences. The whole was surrounded with a high wall. Behind that wall, a building for the administration was erected, and still another wall added which enclosed that building. A prison and detention centre were established there. Before, several dozen prisoners of war inhabited the barracks; now the capacity was set at 1,540 prisoners, 8 cubic metres per person according to the regulations. In practice, the population of the Sluzewiec Prison often exceeded 2,000 inmates. Three double-decker beds were put in small cells, and extra inmates slept on straw mattresses on the floor. After work, the inmates were locked in their cells.

Work occupied most of the prisoners' time. There was no factory in the prison itself; but I dare say it was not by chance that many enterprises employing prisoners soon sprang up in the neighbourhood.

The prison's proper designation is 'Penal Labour Centre for First Offenders', that is, it is a half-open prison. Its inmates should be non-recidivists who still have up to six years of a prison term to serve. At present, the average term still to be served does not exceed two years. But just a few years ago the prison housed men sentenced to six years or longer for petty offences. Attacked in the *Seym Bulletin* (the official government record) in 1987 for the bad situation in prisons, the ex-chief of the prison system put up the following defence:

I believe prisons could and should function normally. But during the 35 years of my work there, I have never witnessed normal functioning. Things go on from one operation or amnesty act to another. . . . I do not want to be misunderstood. I do not intend to criticise the penal policy as it is a result of a definite situation. It follows from the prison staff's experience, however, that policy should be more stable. . . . If we send a man with six years still to serve to a penal labour centre and take him to work outside – and there are 30,000 such inmates – this means that other measures instead of imprisonment might be applied towards them just as well.[8]

Despite this view, however, for many years the prison staff in general backed this highly repressive penal policy, stating emphatically that despite the difficult conditions the prisons would certainly accommodate and employ all newcomers. This was achieved, however, at the expense of prisoners' rights and their conditions of imprisonment.

It was only in recent years that the prison staff realized that although they had no hand in sentencing, they *were* responsible for the atmosphere inside the prison. Two years ago, the Sluzewiec Prison, with its then capacity of 1,540, had 2,500 inmates crammed into it. In its eight barracks, which many years ago were found not worth repairing, and were now ready to be pulled down, men were kept crowded in cells which opened only to let them go to work, and to accept on return. Unsurprisingly, it was very difficult to maintain order in such conditions. The proliferating and irregular penalties, far from bringing improvement, made matters worse. Tensions and deep mutual animosity between guards and inmates could be sensed immediately on entering the prison.

Now, the new attitude to the role of prisons is an example of the changes everywhere in Polish society. The Sluzewiec Prison is a good example of those changes.

I visited the Sluzewiec Prison often over a period of three months, and saw it become a new institution practically every month. Neither the staff nor the management were changed; what changed completely, however, was the atmosphere. It was enough in the Polish conditions to let the staff behave more humanely and most used this opportunity.

Though it is isolated from the world with double walls, the Sluzewiec Prison bears the title of half-open institution. This is because of the categories of its inmates and the fact that they work outside the prison. Today, the half-open character also finds its expression in the relaxation of rules. Such relaxation had already been possible before, but it only occurred with the changed attitude overall towards prisons.

Apart from the above-mentioned category of prisoners (intentional offenders with up to six years still to serve), the prison accommodates all unintentional offenders from Warsaw who were not awaiting trial. Most of them are then sent on to other prisons. Some, however, serve their terms in the Sluzewiec Prison for economic or personal reasons (because of a short sentence or the possibility of maintaining contacts with their families). The general principle, however, is that intentional and unintentional offenders should not be kept together.

Over 70 per cent of inmates are employed outside the prison. They used to work in several dozen, and now work in about a dozen, firms and factories, from building to heavy engineering and metal-lurgical industry to dairies, meat processing plants and clothes factories. Employment of prisoners is profitable for the firms: the Governor stresses that it is only owing to the smaller population of inmates that the number of work-places has reduced. At the begin-ning of 1989, the prison still had nearly 1,000 inmates; in April, there were 800, late in May, 600, and in the first days of July, as few as 500. The only firm on the premises is a Design Office which prepares designs for the prison system, the Ministry of Justice, and the Public Prosecutor's Office. Over twenty prisoners work there. Some also do unpaid work, helping maintain the prison, the kitchen, laundry, library, etc.

A small group of inmates do outwork. It is done in cells and consists of easy and simple (though not always healthy) manual operations, such as pasting envelopes or small wooden elements.

An event that was particularly influential with respect to the changes now taking place was the transfer to Sluzewiec, in 1987, of a special unit for imprisoned drug addicts. The acceptance of a special, much milder, regime for drug addicts as compared with other categories of prisoners is a peculiar feature of the Polish prison system. Such units often employ specialists (psychologists, teachers, sociologists), many of them truly committed and keen actually to help that category of prisoner. It is quite clear that the vigour and determination of the staff of the special ward (a woman psychologist who is head of the ward and one senior sociologist) paved the way to change for the entire Sluzewiec Prison. The begin-nings were not all that easy. The requirements for the new unit were that two selected guards and nobody else should be assigned to the ward; the ward should have a sewage system added; cells should be left unlocked; the inmates should be permitted to wear their own clothes and to garden; the unit head and the senior sociologist should also wear their own civilian clothes and not uniforms; the demand that inmates stand to attention should be abandoned in the case of addicts; they should be permitted to sit or lie down on the bed during the day; in some cases, they should also be permitted to telephone their mothers, and their family and friends should also have the opportunity to telephone them. These are just a few of the long list of demands; the battle for them lasted for months. On the one hand, this demonstrates the extent of restrictions and rules imposed on a Polish prisoner; on the other hand, the fact that they were achieved is an indication of the avalanche of change that has been possible. Recently, only a part of wards beside the special one was open during the day in the Sluzewiec Prison. Today, cells all over the prison remain open daily, and in three wards where the inmates go to work unsupervised by the staff, the cells are also never locked at night. This makes the prisoners' life easier indeed, considering the lack of WCs in the cells. Moreover, contacts with the outside world have been greatly extended. The visit, drastically restricted before to one hour a month and strictly supervised, now lasts up to ten hours outside the prison, at least once a month, such leaves being granted quite often. The family reports at the prison, signs the prisoner out, and undertakes to bring him back after a specified time, but always before 7 p.m., the time of the evening roll-call. What still grates on such occasions is the verbal routine that accompanies these visits, making the families feel they are collecting or registering a parcel rather than a human being. It seems, however, that the staff have also started to realize it little by little. Also, passes of up to five days, granted as privileges, have become widespread. Before, only the selected, 'tested' prisoners could hope to get one; in practice, this applied to those who collaborated with the staff and informed against their fellow inmates.

The special ward for drug addicts seems also to deserve some credit for the general trend to using privileges rather than punishments in maintaining discipline. The value of maintaining the prisoner's contacts with the outside world, through passes and additional visits, has been recognized. When visits outside prison and passes are kept to the minimum, the problems of homosexuality, homosexual rapes, self-mutilations, and other drastic symptoms of prison subculture are present. These phenomena still plague many Polish closed prisons. The staff are still patronizing towards the inmates and treat them contemptuously; it seems, however, that the conditions which make it possible for the staff to humiliate prisoners and treat them as objects have now started to decline little by little in the Sluzewiec prison.

The Governor's recent decision to permit the inmates to have their own television sets in the cells, although they still cannot have their own radio sets, is truly revolutionary in nature. The reason is probably that there is room for one small television set only in a cell now shared by four to six people; and we can easily imagine the effects of all prisoners simultaneously listening to their own radios, each set tuned to a different programme – with ear-phones being both expensive and hard to get in Poland. Besides, the cells have loudspeakers, broadcasting programmes from the prison's own centre, also operated by the inmates. It cannot be denied, however, that underlying the ban on radio sets was the fear that the prisoners might take to listening to Radio Free Europe, still the most popular station in the outside world. But today such a fear is nothing but a relic: it may therefore be expected that the prisoners will be allowed to have their own radio sets any time now.

The inmates still wear the obligatory prison clothes with the institution's stamp visible on the trousers and jacket alike. They also wear such clothes going to work. More and more often, however, they are permitted to wear their own clothes in prison, in winter above all.

The prison has no school, though individual instruction at secondary school level is organized for drug addicts. The remaining prisoners can take vocational training courses, to be a stoker, or cook, for instance. The courses offered are seldom attractive, but at least they fill in the time of those who are willing to train.

The life of the prisoners at Sluzewiec is rather monotonous. They are roused at 5 a.m.; work starts at about 6–7 a.m. and ends at 3.30 or 4 p.m. Back in the prison, they have dinner, then supper, and should be in bed by 9 p.m. According to the regulations, prisoners should have at least eight hours' sleep, which is why the light is switched off in the cells. In theory, the prisoners are free to practise sport or participate in cultural and educational activities between dinner and supper; but I have never noticed any inmates using the prison's volley-ball field. In the small clubs organized in all the huts, daily papers are neatly arranged on tables. They seem to get an occasional dusting for the visitors' sake. Prisoners are permitted to subscribe to papers and journals, but not all of them can afford it, particularly if all they have by way of cash is the remainder left of their wages after the deduction of 70 to 75 per cent for the public purse.[9] What the prison offers are papers such as *Trybuna Ludu* or *Rzeczpospolita*, the official government and party dailies; but the ruling party arouses no particular interest or liking among prisoners. Despite these elements, however, the everyday life in the Sluzewiec Prison has shaken off a lot that was artificial or simply farcical. Admittedly, on noticing a member of the staff, the prisoner still has to spring to his feet, stand to attention and report. However, the titles of talks the staff prepare for the inmates have ceased to feature those strictly ideological subjects whose contents were equally alien to the audience and to the compulsory lecturers.

Meals are still meagre, and hunger remains a serious problem for prisoners. Nowadays, however, the family is at least permitted to treat the inmate to an extra meal during a visit to the prison; this was previously forbidden. Food parcels are allowed more frequently, too.

Gastric ulcers, diseases of the nervous system, and bad teeth are common among prisoners, and cases of lung diseases and mental disorders are growing in number. But health provision is still highly unsatisfactory, though with a much smaller number of prisoners, the inmates now have at least a greater chance of receiving treatment. The Sluzewiec Prison should have fourteen medical officers but this is not the case. Permanently employed are: one general practitioner, one dentist, and one nurse. Specialists, including a dermatologist, a laryngologist, a phthisiologist and a neurologist, are employed part time. According to the Governor, there is no need at present to employ the entire staff of specialists full time.

The Sluzewiec Prison has a total of 200 established posts, the changing size of its population exerting no influence on the number of staff. A half of those posts are taken by the security department, and 20 by education staff. The rest are employed in managing and financial departments, on records, the health service and the administration. The immediate educational needs of inmates should be met by the education staff but it is in their department that the greatest number of vacant posts can be found. The Sluzewiec Prison was not spared the general trend: those who left were the young, well-educated tutors who refused to put up with the omnipotence of the security department and the bad conditions of work. Hence the present solution is to remodel the tasks of the security staff: instead of just guarding and locking doors, the guards are to perform educational functions as well. It is an experiment which may prove successful. With a smaller prison population, anonymity of inmates decreases. Open cells change the quality of the inmates' contacts with guards. The guard is no longer a dictator who decides whether the inmate should be allowed to relieve nature. The two start talking with each other, and the factors which breed mutual suspicion and animosity decrease. This is possible in the Sluzewiec Prison in particular, as the local guards and inmates have quite a number of common interests. The latter are anxious to work outside where they can have many contacts with the ordinary world. The former, instead, want to earn a favourable opinion from their superiors. Each of the parties works for the status and living conditions of the other party. Before, their joint life was based on bullying and hatred: now, this is gradually being replaced by mutual tolerance.

This is just the beginning of a long path. The Sluzewiec Prison is one where in very bad living conditions and with no financial subsidies, attempts are being made at ameliorating the effects of deprivation of liberty, and to make it possible both for the inmates and the guards to behave in a way acceptable in the outer world. This is hardly an easy task since the prison life and rules – those valid at present and those that came into force on 1 October 1989 alike – are simply larded with artificiality: from the obligatory form 'citizen' with which the guards and inmates are to address each other (but which is generally considered offensive, the form 'Mister' being in universal use) – all the way to the preservation of the prisoner's unpaid work and of jobs which, though paid, are nevertheless of no advantage whatever on release and offer no preparation for earning a living even for a few days. Prison remains a world that perverts and desocializes. Moreover, the staff fear it might not be long before the present situation is changed for the worse. How much longer will they be permitted go give prisoners a 'humane' treatment, to aim for, even if not to achieve, a certain 'normality'? What does bring some hope, though – may it not result from our credulity! – is the fact that at present Polish penal policy seems to be fairly stable, and prison conditions are tending gradually to be relaxed not only in Sluzewiec Prison but also in institutions with a stricter regime.

## NOTES

1 In 1956, Polish society protested for the first time against the authorities. As a result, considerable changes were introduced, including the first suspension ever, or at least for some time, of the Stalinist totalitarian methods of government. Further protests took place in 1968, 1970, 1976, 1980–1, 1986 and 1988.

2 See: *System penitencjarny, Stan i wnioski (The Penitentiary System: State and Conclusions)*, a report published for the Minister of Justice, compiled by a team of functionaries of the Central Prison Management and accepted by the Minister of Justice, Warsaw, January 1989.

3 On the use of amnesty in Polish penal policy see: M. Platek (1986) *The Amnesty and Polish Practice*, Vienna.

4 For statistical data on the activities of administration of justice in 1988, see: *Statystyka sadowa i penitencjarna (Court and Penitentiary Statistics)*, January 1989, Warsaw.

5 See: *Biuletyn Sejmu z Komisji Administracji, Spraw Wewnetrznych i Wymiaru Sprawiedliwosci (Seym Bulletin: Proceedings of the Commission of Administration, Internal Affairs and Administration of Justice)*, 21 January 1987, Warsaw. For the statement of the then Director-General of the Prison System see p. 5.

6 See: M. Platek (1987) 'Economic aspects of imprisonment in Poland', unpublished typescript, Oslo-Warsaw; M. Platek, 'Warunkowe zwolnienie a praca skazanych w swietle ustawy i praktyki' ('Conditional release and prisoners' work in the light of law and practice'), in Z. Holda *et al.* (eds) (1985) *Praca skazanych odbywajacych kare pozbawienia wolnosci (The Work of Prisoners)*, Lublin, pp. 90–103.

7 As a result of strikes which the working classes organized in 1980, the first independent trade union of Polish employees, 'Solidarity', was established in August 1980.

8 *Seym Bulletin*, op.cit., pp. 6–7.

9 If the prisoner is obliged to pay maintenance, the reduction is limited to 25 per cent, and the bulk of his salary paid in as maintenance.

*Chapter Four*

# HELDERSTROOM PRISON, SOUTH AFRICA

## *DIRK VAN ZYL SMIT*

### I

> The writer begs his reader to excuse the frequent egotisms which
> he does not know how to avoid, without using circumlocutions
> that might have been more disgusting. (Howard 1929: xxii)

Thus wrote John Howard in 1777 in the introduction to *The State of
the Prisons*. The particular circumstances of South Africa require a
similar indulgence from the reader.

In late July 1989 I applied to the South African prison authorities
in Pretoria for permission to visit a prison for adult males so that I
could respond to an invitation from the Howard League to describe
such a prison. I chose Helderstroom Prison simply because it was a
prison I had not been shown before and I knew that it was not one
to which visitors are usually taken. After relatively uncomplicated
negotiations the prison authorities agreed to my request. During my
two visits to Helderstroom the authorities answered my questions
with exemplary patience. I was allowed to speak freely to junior
members of the prison service and to prisoners of my choice. However, the practical problems of lack of privacy and of being an
'outsider', and so probably perceived as associated with the authorities, made it hard to achieve adequate rapport with the prisoners.
Subsequently, in order to verify my impressions, I also interviewed a
prisoner who had recently been released from Helderstroom.

Although they occasionally expressed some anxiety about what I
might say, the prison authorities did not put any pressure on me to
submit my account to them prior to publication. Such pressure
might have been expected as the South African Prisons Act contains
severe restrictions on the publication of 'false' information about

prisons or prisoners. If such information is published the onus is on the publisher to show that he or she took reasonable steps prior to publication to ensure the accuracy of the report.[1] Failure to meet these requirements can result, on conviction, in a prison sentence of up to two years and a substantial fine.[2] For many years the effect of this penal provision, which was broadly interpreted by the courts, was to inhibit drastically all reporting on South African prisons. In 1984, however, the Prisons Service came to an arrangement with the major newspaper publishers: the authorities would regard the requirements of the Act as having been met if the newspapers undertook to submit all reports to them before publication and published, with equal prominence, any comments that the Prisons Service might wish to make (Stuart 1986). At the same time restrictions were lifted on at least some of the numerous critical accounts of South African prisons.[3]

Commentators outside the national press are not covered by the 'arrangement', which, in any event, is of doubtful legal status. The account which follows was not shown to the Prisons Service before submission for publication although, inevitably, much of the information was in any case obtained from official sources. I have reported as accurately as I could. The provisions of the Prisons Act played no part in my decisions on what to include or omit. The views expressed are my own and quite clearly not those of the Prisons Service.

## II

Imprisonment is a key element in the system of social control in South Africa. This is true in the general sense that a very high proportion of the total population of the Republic of South Africa is incarcerated, either awaiting trial or as sentenced prisoners. Thus, the most recent *Report of the Department of Justice* reveals that there were 110,481 prisoners on 30 June 1988 (Department of Justice 1988: 142–3). Of these, 90,485 were sentenced prisoners. A further unknown number of prisoners awaiting trial are detained in police cells and thus fall outside the ambit, and the statistics, of the Prisons Service. On 30 June 1988 there were, according to the figures provided by the service, 306 persons per 100,000 of the officially estimated population of the Republic of South Africa in custody as sentenced prisoners. The ratio for all persons in prison on the same date was 373 per 100,000.[4]

The sentence of imprisonment appears to be imposed fairly readily. There are no precise statistics but the *Report of the Central Statistical Services* for 1 July 1986 to 30 June 1987 reveals that 380,094 people were convicted by South African courts. According to the *Report of the Department of Justice* for the same period 180,453 persons were admitted to prison as sentenced offenders. From these figures it can be deduced that 47 per cent of offenders sentenced by the courts spent some time in prison. Whether they were sentenced without an option, or went to prison because they could not afford to pay fines, is not clear.

In South Africa prisoners are classified as 'White' (people of European origin), 'Asian' (people from the Indian subcontinent), 'Black' (people of pure African descent) or 'Coloured' (people of mixed race). These classifications, which are refined beyond what is indicated in the parentheses, are offensive to many South Africans, because they provide the basis for racial discrimination. In particular, it is more acceptable to use the term 'Black' for any South African not classified as 'White'. However, as will become apparent, official classification continues to play an important part in the operation of the prison system. These figures reveal remarkable differences in the proportion of prisoners from each racial category. On 30 June 1988 the figure per 100,000 for 'Whites' was 92 and for 'Asians' 78. In contrast, the ratio for 'Blacks' (Africans) was 381 and for 'Coloureds', 851 per 100,000.[5]

In South Africa imprisonment also plays a vital part in what has been called 'regime maintenance' (Potts 1984). A variety of 'extraordinary provisions'[6] allows for detention without trial. These range from preventive detention,[7] detention for interrogation[8] and the detention of witnesses[9] under the permanent security legislation, and to the detention of reluctant informers under the legislation relating to prohibited drugs.[10] Such detention may be for indeterminate periods and is only subject to very restricted controls on the abuse of state power. In addition, a State of Emergency was declared in some parts of South Africa on 21 July 1985.[11] Since 12 June 1986 a State of Emergency has been in force throughout South Africa.[12] Under the extraordinary Emergency powers any member of the police force, the military or even the Prisons Service has the power

71

to arrest and detain.[13] Detention, which may be either preventive or for interrogation, is virtually indefinite (subject only to the annual renewal of the Emergency) and subject to no effective judicial control.[14]

The various extraordinary provisions make it difficult to gain a full statistical picture of the number of people actually incarcerated in South Africa. Those held in prison under the permanent security legislation and of the legislation relating to drugs are listed separately in the official prison statistics (Department of Justice 1988: 142–3), but those 'temporarily' detained in police cells are not recorded. Emergency detainees in prison are included along with prisoners awaiting trial and no accurate figures for them are available. It is estimated that since the first State of Emergency in 1985, up to 30,000 people may have been detained under the emergency provisions (*South*, 8 June 1989). At the time of writing, relatively few people are being held under the State of Emergency.[15] However, many ex-detainees have been placed under such draconian restrictions that they are under virtual house arrest and thus removed from political and community life.[16]

The South African prison system is a centralized bureaucracy organized on quasi-military lines. Prisons Service policy is determined centrally and applied throughout the country. The military-style structure is strongly hierarchical and led by a Commissioner of Prisons who holds the rank of Lieutenant-General. As officer in charge of the Prisons Service, the Commissioner of Prisons is answerable to the Director-General of Justice, who is the civil service head of the Department of Justice into which the Prisons Service falls, and the Minister of Justice who is the political head of the department. The Prisons Service is divided into four regions amongst which 28 prisons commands (or groups) and 206 separate prisons are distributed. All follow strictly the guide-lines laid down from the central authority.

The 206 prisons vary from small local gaols to large prisons which serve the metropolitan areas and which may have more than 3,000 inmates. Twelve of them are rated as exclusively maximum security prisons, but many of the remaining 'medium' prisons also house prisoners who are rated as a maximum security risk. Minimum security prisons are still at the stage of the drawing board. There are a few specialized prisons for adult males. These include 16 prison farms. At 6 prisons there are 'production workshops', at 8 prisons 'building training centres' and 26 prisons have 'maintenance workshops'. The prison population as a whole is relatively stable. Over the past decade the number of short-term sentences has declined, probably as a result of the demise of influx control on 'Blacks' (Africans). However, the number of long-term prisoners has increased. On 20 January 1989, 64 per cent of all prisoners (69,666 persons) were serving sentences of two years or longer (*Hansard* 1989).

The prisons system has long struggled to provide accommodation for all these prisoners. On 30 June 1988 it could house 83,668 prisoners and was thus 32 per cent overcrowded (Department of Justice 1988: 67). In spite of a policy of reallocating prisoners in order to alleviate gross overcrowding in a particular area, individual prisons are still often much more crowded than the national norm. The staff:prisoner ratio in the service as a whole on 30 June 1988 was 1 staff member to 5.5 prisoners. This figure is an underestimate of the actual ratio at individual prisons as it includes the central administrative staff. Nevertheless the relatively high prisoner:staff ratio explains, at least in part, why the total cost per prisoner was only R13.28 (£3.04) per prisoner per day at the end of March 1988 (Department of Justice 1988: 108 and *passim*).

## III

The Helderstroom prison complex is one of the sixteen prison farms in the South African prison system. It was established in 1971 and is situated on 1,000 hectares of prime agricultural land, about 120 km from Cape Town. The prison farm is relatively isolated, at the end of a 5 km stretch of unsurfaced road and about 30 km from the two nearest towns of Caledon and Villiersdorp.

The first impression is of a neat modern village built on a hill and clustered around two larger structures. Closer inspection reveals two separate, virtually identical prisons a few hundred metres apart. These are Helderstroom Maximum Security Prison and Helderstroom Medium Security Prison (referred to as 'maximum' and 'medium' respectively). On both the south and the north side of the hill are rows of staff housing. On the northern side live the 182 'White' members of staff and the southern side houses most of the 150 'Coloured' staff members. All except ten of the 332 members of the Prisons Service live permanently on the prison farm.

On 9 August 1989 the two prisons together housed 2,397 prisoners, 1,300 of these in the medium security prison and the remaining 1,097 in the maximum security prison. Helderstroom, as a whole, had a staff:prisoner ratio of one staff member to 7.2 prisoners. All of the prisoners were sentenced and were serving sentences of longer than two years for 'ordinary' common law crimes. Helderstroom is not an admission centre and all prisoners had been referred from other prisons. They were all 'Coloured' males and all adult, except for some 60 juveniles (under the age of 21) in a separate section of 'medium'. It was explained that all the 'Black' (African) prisoners under the jurisdiction of the prison command, of which Helderstroom forms part, were held at a similar prison some 80 km away, so that when interpreters were required they could be provided at a central point. It was not thought necessary to explain the absence of 'White' prisoners. In a sense, therefore, the racial segregation was even more rigorous than is required by the Prisons Act, the legislation that provides the legal framework for the South African prison system. Section 23 (1) of the Prisons Act lays down that

> (b) as far as possible, white and non-white prisoners shall be detained in separate parts thereof and in such manner as to prevent white and non-white prisoners from being within view of each other; and
> (c) wherever practicable, non-white prisoners of different races shall be separated.

Apart from the racial criteria and the length of sentence there did not appear to be any reason why particular prisoners were being kept at Helderstroom. No prisoners convicted of crimes against the security of the state (sentenced political prisoners) were at Helderstroom, although prison officers recalled that some years previously a group of 75 such 'Black' (African) prisoners had been held there. Nor were there any emergency or security detainees. However, the State of Emergency had not left Helderstroom unscathed. Some time before, a maximum security section of a prison in a neighbouring command had been cleared entirely to make room for Emergency detainees and some of these prisoners had been transferred to Helderstroom. Since then things had returned to 'normal'. The occupancy rate on 9 August could therefore not be regarded as abnormal. On that day the medium and maximum prisons were overcrowded by 72 and 86 per cent respectively. It is necessary to explain what these rates mean. The norms adopted by the Prisons Service allow 3.334 sq. m per prisoner in a communal cell and 5.5 sq. m per single cell. 'Air space' should be 4.25 cu. m per prisoner. These norms, the service argues, are generous, given that most prisoners spend a large period of time each day outside their cells.

In practical terms overcrowding at the level recorded in Helderstroom maximum has severe effects, particularly where the majority of prisoners are held in communal cells. At Helderstroom maximum there was officially room for 590 prisoners. This would mean that if the population was equally distributed the occupancy rate of the communal cells was 253 per cent. During my second visit on 16 August, however, it was explained to me that for some time a number of prisoners had been housed in the second dining area. I was told that on 9 August, 171 prisoners were accommodated in the dining area which measures 23 m by 15 m. (My information was that they had to roll up all their bedding and stow their possessions as this area was still used for meals from 7.15 a.m. onwards.) The result was that the remaining 668 prisoners were divided amongst 15 communal cells. This would mean that, if an optimum distribution was achieved, there were 44.5 prisoners per cell. The size of these cells, excluding the ablution area, was approximately 15 m x 5 m. In other words, in a cell with 45 occupants, each prisoner had only 1.67 sq. m of floor space.

As far as physical structure, the maximum and medium buildings were substantially identical in design. Official policy is not to differentiate architecturally between these two types. Similarly, treatment of higher security risks in the maximum prison is intended to be substantially the same as in the medium prison. Under current policy the privilege-category of a prisoner is not determined by his security rating. Prisoners of all the privilege-categories are found in both prisons. Those with the same ratings are housed together in particular cells or parts of each prison.

At Helderstroom the joint headquarters was at the medium prison, as were the offices of the welfare and employment officers, the hospital and the morgue. The medium prison could accommodate slightly more prisoners than the maximum because it included fewer single cells. My inspection of physical conditions was made mostly in the maximum security prison but, unless exception is made, my observations could apply to both prisons.

I was struck by how clean the prisons were and how well the surroundings had been cared for. The maximum prison had been prepared for a special inspection (certainly not something that I requested or wanted!) and in the medium prison the normal week-day routine was left uninterrupted.

Elaborate, almost bizarre preparations had been made for the inspection on 9 August of the communal cells in the maximum. Here the prisoners all sleep on the floor. (Only the prisoners in the medium prison sleep on beds.) Their bedding, thin mats and blankets, had been lightly rolled and twisted into most complicated forms and then decorated with highly coloured bits of wool. In between the bedding rolls paths had been made with crinkled paper and the intervening area strewn with what looked like confetti. The walls too were decorated with murals, often of nineteenth-century Boer generals or twentieth-century political leaders. These too were festooned with streamers. The total effect was of a deserted Christmas party which had turned into a surrealist nightmare. This effect was heightened by a choir which had been located in a nearby stairwell and which boomed out echoing revivalist anthems throughout my 'tour' of these cells.

One of the more detailed observations which I could make, apart from the size of the cells and how crowded they must be, was the total lack of privacy and personal space. Since there are no fixed beds the whole room has to be arranged daily. This means that prisoners are limited to one small locker each. I estimated each locker to be only 0.2 cu. m in size. Even these lack permanence. Thus in a cell designed for, say, twenty-five inmates there would be twenty-five lockers. The additional twenty or so prisoners would have to put their few personal possessions into portable plastic boxes of approximately the same size as the 'permanent' lockers. For the purposes of the tour these boxes were bundled into a corner or into the bathroom area and covered with a blanket.

The ablution facilities in the communal cells were very limited. Each cell had a single toilet, a wash basin and three showers to be shared by forty-five prisoners. The toilet was constructed in such a way that a prisoner using it would be screened from the body of the communal cells but not from others using the ablution area.

Outside these communal cells there was little about the physical surroundings to inspire comment. The sick bays in both prisons appeared clean and well equipped. The same applied to the kitchens, the library and to the classroom that I saw. A noticeable feature of the dining areas was that they were entirely bare. The prisoners have to squat on the concrete and eat their food with spoons from single bowls.

A prime feature of the prison buildings was the two large quadrangles in each prison. They are surrounded on all sides by the double-storey buildings of the prison. They measure approximately 50 m by 45 m and have concrete surfaces. A tennis court was the only visible recreational feature in the quadrangle which I observed most closely.

Outside the two prison buildings there is little at Helderstroom to distinguish it physically from an efficient mixed farm. There are several hectares of planted pasturage, grazed by sheep and cows. There are workshops for the maintenance of farming and prison equipment. There are small building operations. There are batteries of chickens and sheds filled with pigsties, which make up the factory-farming aspects of the whole enterprise. Along the banks of the picturesquely named Riviersonderend (river without end), below the hill on which the prison buildings and staff housing are situated, there are intensively cultivated fields where several varieties of vegetables are grown.

## IV

A typical routine on a weekday at Helderstroom would be as follows: Prisoners are woken at 5.30 a.m. and the cells are unlocked at 7.00 a.m. (In the summer the medium prison is unlocked at 6.30 a.m.) Firearms are issued to the warders who take prisoners to work outside the prison buildings. The warders inside are all unarmed. The prisoners are mustered in the quadrangle for scripture reading and prayers. Breakfast is taken at 7.10 a.m. The work teams are then marched out at 7.30 a.m. Those who remain behind take part in educational programmes, attend confirmation classes, go to the library, meet social workers or the doctor, or participate in 'recreational activities' in the quadrangle. Those who work outside the prison take lunch at their stations. Inside, lunch is eaten between 11.00 and 11.30 a.m. and the prisoners are then locked in their cells until 2.00 p.m. After that they may resume the activities of the morning. At 4.00 p.m. the prisoners who have been working outside return and are all searched as a matter of routine. Supper is taken between 4.00 and 4.20 p.m. At 5.00 p.m. prisoners are locked in their cells until the next morning. At 5.15 p.m. most of the prison staff go off duty. Lights in the cells are put off in the medium prison at 8.30 p.m. In maximum they remain on all night. That, simply, is the structure of the day but almost every aspect of this routine has to be detailed and qualified if one is to understand what it means in practice.

A careful analysis of the numbers of prisoners marched out to work on 9 August shows that relatively few were involved in farming activities. Thus in the medium prison, 836, or 64 per cent, of the prisoners were employed but only 321 of them worked on tasks which could be identified with the farming activities of the prison. In the maximum prison the picture was even less rosy. The number employed was 341, 31 per cent of the total. However, none of them were employed in agriculture. (More than two-thirds of those employed from maximum were working on the construction of a new soccer field.) If the total population of prisoners at Helderstroom is taken together it can be seen that only 13 per cent of all the prisoners were actually employed in agriculture.

From the perspective of rehabilitative 'treatment' and 'training (of prisoners) in habits of industry and labour',[17] which together form an important part of the statutory functions of the Prisons Service, doubts can be raised about the efficacy of farm labour. Most of the prisoners were used to perform the most menial tasks. Only a few were involved in activities such as sheep-shearing, which require more than a modicum of skill. The same was true of the maintenance workshops where, at best, thirty prisoners were involved in activities which required some knowledge of a trade. Indeed, broader questions could be asked about the whole agricultural thrust of the prison, for it seemed as if many, perhaps a majority of the prisoners, were from the greater Cape Town urban area and were unlikely ever to find, or wish to find, employment in agriculture. What the Helderstroom farm does effectively, according to official accounts, is produce enough meat, vegetables and dairy products to make the Helderstroom prisons and also the smaller local prison in Caledon self-sufficient in these respects. (Prison farm produce is not sold on the open market.)

On might have expected that the shortcomings of the work pro-gramme would be compensated for by the other activities available to prisoners who were not being punished by being held in solitary confinement. Some schooling was offered during the day, to 120 prisoners in maximum and 90 in medium. Prisoners who wished to participate in a literacy programme were allocated to one com-munal cell in each prison, so that they could study in the evenings. However, one cell was not sufficient to meet the demand. However, even if those who attended school during the day were added to those who worked outside, the fact remained that the majority of those detained in maximum were unemployed and unoccupied during the day. On the occasion of my visit I found almost 400 prisoners in a single quadrangle (of 2,250 sq. m) in maximum, where they spent their time while others worked. Two were playing tennis in a blustering wind. The others appeared merely to be standing about. I was told by a prisoner who was the enthusiastic chairman of the recreational committee that prisoners also play darts, kerrim (a board game), volley-ball (on the tennis court) and Rugby (on an outside pitch) over the weekends. There is reason for scepticism over whether the large mass of prisoners were actively involved in these activities.

Most of the specialized services offered by the prisons are also made available to prisoners during the morning and afternoon work periods. Perhaps most prominent amongst these are medical ser-vices. Each prison has its own medical orderlies and clinics. The orderlies fulfil first aid functions and also perform tasks such as weighing prisoners and dispensing prescribed medicine from a trolley which is wheeled to the dining areas in the morning and evening. A doctor, the district surgeon of the nearest town (Caledon), who is a medical practitioner in government employ, visits each of the two prisons once a week to attend to prisoners who have reported sick. He sees about seventy to eighty patients in the course of the morning and also the few serious cases which might be referred from the other prison. There is no doctor available at short notice. In emergencies the ambulance at the prison is used to take seriously ill prisoners to Caledon Hospital, where they are treated by qualified personnel. There are no psychologists at Helder-stroom. The prison psychologist from the command headquarters some 80 km away visits at most once a fortnight.

Prisoners' needs for social services are supposed to be met by social workers employed by the Prisons Service. The centralized social work section at Helderstroom has a staff of six, of whom three are qualified social workers. In theory therefore they each have enormous case-loads. However, it appears as if, apart from completing essential forms, they only help when requested. Only those who are regarded as susceptible to treatment (*behandelingsvatbaar*) are attended to throughout their stay in prison. However, all prisoner are 'prepared for release' by the social workers. What this entails did not become clear to me.

As far as could be ascertained, the daily routine met the prisoners' basic needs. Clothing appeared to be adequate. On my second visit on 16 August, a cold and rainy winter morning, the prisoners appeared to be dressed reasonably warmly in a variety of khaki clothes. Some had jackets but the issue of these has apparently been discontinued. Those who had to go out were issued with waterproof capes. The food that I saw appeared adequate and none of the prisoners obviously starved, but I did not study a full menu. The gap from the supper to breakfast is excessively long (particularly on weekends when 'supper' is at 3.15 p.m.). I also noticed on 9 August that the actual cooking of the supper was completed by mid-morning, as the midday meal consisted only of sandwiches. However, I was told that prisoners may take some of the bread from supper with them to their cells.

There are some variations of the daily routine. On rainy days only a few prisoners go out to work and most are simply kept in their cells. I was told that over weekends only a very limited number of prisoners go out to perform essential services. Others may be involved in Rugby or soccer matches on Saturday mornings or (non-compulsory) church parades on a Sunday. In the afternoons they all remain in the quadrangles between 2.00 p.m. and supper at 3.15 p.m. Most of the prison staff go off duty at 4.00 p.m. over the weekends.

Prisoners in the single cells at maximum are regarded as the 'hardest cases' and their routines are somewhat restricted. They do not work outside the prison or attend classes. They take exercise in a quadrangle away from the prisoners in the communal cells. They are divided into two groups of about one hundred which, in order to separate warring factions, are not allowed to exercise simultaneously. Although not subject to a 'punishment' regime, their time in the open is in effect only 50 per cent of that of other prisoners.

The routine of prisoners sentenced to solitary confinement in punishment cells (to which they may be sentenced by an officer's court) is also severely restricted. They are allowed only the two statutory half-hour exercise periods per day in a separate, smaller quadrangle of 10 m by 20 m. The regime in the punishment cell may include periods of 'reduced diet' (half the daily intake) and 'spare diet' which consists of only 200 gm of maize meal twice daily, boiled in water without salt and 15 gm of soup powder boiled in 530 ml of water once daily.[18] I was told that this spare diet is weighed meticulously. Apart from isolation and dietary punishments an officer's court may sentence male prisoners under the age of 40 years to corporal punishment. I did not investigate this aspect thoroughly, but was told that at Helderstroom corporal punishment was imposed about twice a month, in the prison as a whole.

## V

The dangers of total estrangement from the outside world are particularly severe in as isolated a prison as Helderstroom. They exist not only for the prisoners but also for the staff who live in a separate community away from the influence of towns and villages. However, staff members assured me that they had adequate contact with the surrounding farmers and with the townspeople of Caledon, to which the children are bused to school each day. Many of the staff had grown up in villages and on farms and professed a preference for a quiet life.

From the prisoners' point of view the privilege system is an important determinant of how much contact they are allowed with the outside world. All the prisoners at Helderstroom are in the privilege-categories 2, 3 and 4 of the four possible 'notches' in the system. (Category 1, the lowest category, is apparently only used for recently admitted prisoners.) This means that they are entitled to receive and send 20, 30 or 40 letters per year depending on their privilege category. Category 4 prisoners may also receive a daily newspaper. All this communication is strictly censored and prisoners are specifically prohibited from expressing complaints about prison conditions in their correspondence. In practice the prisoners at Helderstroom do not subscribe to newspapers. (I was told that only the sentenced 'political' prisoners who had been held there earlier, had done so.) Prisoners are allowed to hear uncensored news bulletins on the state-controlled radio. Category 4 prisoners are also allowed, once in a few days, to watch videos on television sets brought to their cells. All prisoners at Helderstroom are allowed access to the library. In practice utilization of the library is relatively low. Less than one book per prisoner per month is borrowed in maximum and two per prisoner in medium. An unknown percentage of the prisoners is illiterate.

Visits are also allowed. A category 2 prisoner may receive twenty 30-minute visits a year while a category 4 prisoner may be visited 30 times annually for up to 40 minutes. Such visits are tightly controlled. Only category 4 prisoners are allowed contact visits and a warder is always present. There is no provision for conjugal visits. The distance of Helderstroom from the metropolitan area of Cape Town inhibits visiting severely. However, NICRO (the charity concerned with the welfare of offenders) has organized a bus service which runs from Cape Town to Helderstroom on two Sundays a month. Isolation remains a problem. I spoke to a prisoner serving a consecutive sentence of 48 years in total for multiple armed robberies (an exceptional sentence by South African standards), who had not been visited for a year and whose family, he said, ignored all his correspondence.

Nothing concrete could be established about the reconviction rates of the prisoners at Helderstroom. This must handicap the Institutional Committee which serves both prisons and which is responsible for calculating projected dates on which prisoners can be released either unconditionally (that is, if they do not forfeit the remission which they are provisionally allocated on admission), or conditionally on parole. The Institutional Committee makes recommendations about release to a higher authority and also attends to the reclassification of prisoners. The impression with which I was left was that, in the absence of information on likely reconviction rates or other statistical projections, the Institutional Committee followed bureaucratic guide-lines very closely.

## VI

The attitudes of staff and prisoners to each other and to themselves reflect in many ways the social and even linguistic structures of the society as a whole. Prison life in South Africa throughout most of this century has been dominated by prison gangs which exist in virtually all prisons. Helderstroom is no exception and the prisoners confirmed that they either were or had been members of prison gangs. In particular, those with whom I spoke (not necessarily a representative sample) claimed membership of the '28' gang, a gang whose activities were focused on the procurement of catamites in prison. (Sodomy is a major problem for both the authorities and the prisoners at Helderstroom. Several of the prisoners in the single cells at Helderstroom asked to be put there for protection from homosexual assaults. Prisoners are warned against AIDS, but not issued with condoms.) Both prisoners and staff emphasized, though, that gang activity had decreased and that, particularly in the medium prison, the gangs did not hold sway to the same extent as they had done in the past. This was supported by the fact that, unlike several other prisons in the region, there had not been a gang murder at Helderstroom in recent years.

The attitudes of the staff as a group are also interesting. In many ways the staff facilities and the inter-personal relationships reflect the apartheid structures of a small South African town. The separate residential areas which I have described are mirrored in separate messes and clubs and even in the separate buses that take the children to their segregated schools in the nearest town. The only mixing between racial groups at a social level appears to be a joint Rugby team. Yet, at the official level, there have been changes. The chief social worker and the full-time chairman of the Institutional Committee are both 'Coloured' and both hold the rank of captain. As far as I could observe, they are accorded the formal respect due to their rank. (They outranked most other prison staff members. In the military hierarchy of the Prisons Service the officer in charge of the whole Helderstroom complex has the rank of lieutenant-colonel and the heads of the medium and maximum prisons are both majors.) The prisoners did not perceive a great difference between the attitudes of 'White' and 'Coloured' staff.

The question of the relationship of the staff to the prisoners is complex. The policy of the Prisons Service is that prisoners of all races should be treated equally and some steps have been taken to remove racially discriminatory provisions from prison legislation. However, the formal policy of separate but equal treatment has not been (and probably can never be) fully implemented. To take a single example, all 'White' prisoners sleep in beds, while this 'privilege' is only being extended selectively to those prisoners not classified as 'White'. Moreover, the social distance between 'White' staff and prisoners is great. This reflects itself in the language. Although there is a common language (Afrikaans is the mother tongue of probably well over 90 per cent of both staff and prisoners at Helderstroom), it is spoken very differently by prisoners and staff. Amongst themselves the former speak a dialect which has developed in the gang context. Towards authority prisoners attempt to speak a more 'acceptable' form of Afrikaans. Like French, Afrikaans has a formal and informal second person pronoun. As a matter of course staff would address prisoners with the informal *jy* (*tu* in French), but would not accept being spoken to by a prisoner in that way. Prisoners tend to use circumlocutions to avoid the second person form. Officially, prisoners should address the members of the service by the ranks, 'warder', 'sergeant', 'major', etc, but the more obsequious forms of 'chief', 'baas' (boss) and 'oubaas' (old boss) have not died out.

## VII

What, one wonders, would John Howard have made of Helderstroom? He might well have been impressed by the cleanliness, by the situation of the prison, by the prison garb and, perhaps, by the food. Yet he would have found much to criticize. Foremost would undoubtedly have been the accommodation. There is simply not enough space at Helderstroom to accommodate all the inmates adequately, let alone to meet Howard's ideal of 'so many small rooms or cabins that each criminal may sleep alone' (Howard 1929: 21). A space of 1.67 sq. m to lay down a thin mat amongst forty-five others is not acceptable by any standards. The lack of privacy in general is extreme. The meals, even if sufficiently nourishing, are taken in the most congested and undignified circumstances imaginable: six hundred prisoners are crouched tightly together back to back in two rooms on the concrete floor of a dining area which is so constricted that only a couple of rows of prisoners can move simultaneously. In spite of its overcrowding, Helderstroom does not appear to be a particularly harsh prison by South African standards. Gang killings and escapes were both less prevalent than elsewhere. Ironically, some prisoners regarded it as desirable because of its 'better facilities'.

What Helderstroom illustrates is the scope of the pressures facing the South African system. The numbers simply overwhelm any serious efforts at the rehabilitation of prisoners. The prison officers are reduced to mere turnkeys, concentrating on containing rather than training prisoners. This is not to say that more could not be done to make this containment more humane. A view of prisoners as fellow citizens whose human rights are to be respected might be more effective than the current attitude: paternalism combined with a conception of prisoners as very different creatures. Changes in the wider South African policy leading to the full abolition of segregation might result in such a shift in attitude. However, the more fundamental problem of limited resources will remain. If the current high proportion of the steadily growing South African population continues to be imprisoned, no future South African government will be able to provide the facilities necessary for the rehabilitative training of prisoners, or even for their detention under humane conditions.

## NOTES

1 Section 44 (1)(f) of the Prisons Act 8 of 1959.
2 Section 44 (1) of the Prisons Act 8 of 1959.
3 Hugh Lewin's *Bandiet* (1976), Harmondsworth: Penguin, is now available in South Africa after having been prohibited for many years. Breyten Breytenbach's *The True Confessions of an Albino Terrorist* (1984), Johannesburg: Taurus, has been freely available in South Africa since its publication.
   Some attempt was made to restrict the distribution of the doctoral thesis of J. Mihalik (*Gevangenisstraf: Die Noodsaaklikheid vir Alternatiewe Strawwe* (1986) (unpublished LLD thesis, Pretoria: University of South Africa), because of the inaccuracies which it is alleged to contain, but Mihalik has subsequently published on aspects of his work in the respected *South African Law Journal:* J. Mihalik (1988) 'Executive manipulation of prison sentences: has the sentencing authority moved to the executive?' *SALJ* 105: 494–518, and J. Mihalik (1989) '"The taming

of the bad, or Unspeakable Cruelty"? – prison disciplinary offences', *SALJ* 106: 319–38.

A much wider interest in prison law has emerged in recent years. Much of the writing is highly critical of the way the courts have developed South African prison law. See, for example, J.H. van Rooyen (1981) 'Aspekte van reg om geregtigheid met betrekking tot gevangenes', *Tydskrif vir Hedendaagse Romeins-Hollandse Reg* 44: 17, and D. van Zyl Smit (1987) '"Normal" prisons in an "abnormal" society?' *Criminal Justice Ethics* 6: 37–51 and the sources cited there.

The 'scientific' literature on prison conditions is smaller. However, an 'outside' researcher was allowed to make a comprehensive study of prison gangs in the early 1980s. After some hesitation this was published in 1984 (J.M. Lotter and W.J. Schurink (1984) *Gevangenisbendes: 'n Ondersoek met spesiale verwysing na nommerbendes onder Kleurling gevangenes*, Pretoria: HSRC). A very flattering account of the South African prison system was produced by a visiting Swiss criminologist, W.T. Haesler (1986) ('Sudafrikanischer Strafvollzug. Eindrucke einer Studienreise im September/Oktober 1984', *Zeitschrift für Strafvollzug und Straffalligenhilfe* 35: 11–17). In my view this account is somewhat superficial (see D. van Zyl Smit (1986) 'Nochmals: Sudafrikanischer Strafvollzug', *Zeitschrift für Strafvollzug und Straffalligenhilfe* 35: 280–4).

Apart from the material on 'ordinary' imprisonment there is also a large body of legal and sociological literature on detention without trial. See D. Foster, D. Davis and D. Sandler (1987) *Detention and Torture in South Africa*, Cape Town: David Philip, and the sources cited there.

4 These figures should be treated with some caution. The ratios might be misleadingly high because the official population estimate of 29,617,000 for June 1988 is held by some demographers to be a drastic underestimate of the real population. It should also be noted that the figures refer to the Republic of South Africa. They thus exclude the populations of the 'independent' national states of Transkei, Ciskei, Venda and Bophuthatswana. It is also not clear whether offenders from these countries are being held in South African prisons.

5 Calculated on the basis of information in the *Annual Report*: 142, and official estimates of population on 30 June 1988.

6 A distinction can be drawn in South Africa between ordinary procedural rules which, broadly speaking, meet procedural due process requirements and which are designed to deal with 'conventional crime' on the one hand, and, on the other hand, a parallel body of drastic or extraordinary provisions which do not meet the most elementary standards of the rule of law.

7 Sections 28 and 50 of the Internal Security Act 74 of 1982.

8 Section 29 of the Internal Security Act 74 of 1982.

9 Section 31 of the Internal Security Act 74 of 1982; cf. also section 185 of the Criminal Procedure Act 51 of 1977, which provides for the detention of witnesses in cases involving serious common law offences.

10 Section 13 of the Abuse of Dependence-producing Substances and Rehabilitation Centres Act 41 of 1971.
11 Proclamation R121 of 1985 under the Public Safety Act 3 of 1953.
12 Proclamation R109 of 1986; the State of Emergency has been renewed annually as required by the Public Safety Act. See Proc R95 of 11 June 1987, Proc R96 of 10 June 1988, and Proc R85 of 9 June 1989.
13 Reg 3(1) read with reg 1 (definitions) of the 'Emergency Security regulations' Proc R86 of 9 June 1989.
14 Reg 3: a large body of case law and comment on these provisions has grown up in the past few years. For an overview, see E. Mureinik (1989) 'Pursuing principle: the Appellate Division and review under the State of Emergency', *South African Journal of Human Rights* 5: 60–72.
15 According to The Human Rights Commission more than 200 people are being held without trial in the Republic of South Africa. These include at least 53 people held under the Emergency Regulations, *Weekly Mail*, 25 August 1989.
16 The Human Rights Commission documented 551 restricted persons in June 1989. It estimated that up to 900 could have been restricted, *Weekly Mail*, 30 June 1989.
17 Section 2(2)(b) of the Prisons Act.
18 Section 54(2)(f) of the Prisons Act read with prison reg 101.

## REFERENCES

Department of Justice (1988) *Report of the Department of Justice for the Republic of South Africa for the period 1 July 1987 to 30 June 1988* (referred to as the *Annual Report*).

Hansard (1989) House of Assembly Debates, Questions and Replies col. 856, 26 April.

Howard, J. (1929) *The State of the Prisons*, Everyman's Library, London: J.M. Dent.

Potts, L.W. (1984) 'Custodial detention and regime maintenance in the Republic of South Africa', *New England Journal of Civil and Criminal Confinement* 10: 301–52.

Stuart, K. (1986) *The Newspaperman's Guide to the Law*, Durban: Butterworth.

# Chapter Five

# BREDA PRISON, HOLLAND

*From water cell to container cell – the state of
the Dutch prison*

## ANTON M. VAN KALMTHOUT AND DIRK VAN DER LANDEN

### THE DUTCH PENAL CLIMATE: REPUTATION AND REALITY

#### *1595: the water cell*

For centuries, the Dutch prison system has had the reputation of
being progressive, moderate and humane. This reputation dates
back to 1595, in which year a men's house of detention was opened
in a former monastery in Amsterdam. This was followed two years
later by the so-called 'spinning house' for women. Differentiation
was completed in 1603 by the establishment of a special correctional
institution for youthful delinquents. These initiatives put into practice the idea developed by Coornhert (1587) and other progressive
humanists in the second half of the sixteenth century that the
punishment and treatment of criminals should not primarily serve
as a deterrent and means of putting them out of the way, but rather
as a means towards reform and education.[1] These aims were to be
achieved through hard physical labour, religious education and
strict discipline. In the 'Rasphouse', two inmates were required to
rasp at least 600 kg of wood per week, an activity that was stimulated
by frequent corporal punishment.[2] This house of detention enjoyed
international fame. In the first place, the regime with its underlying
penitentiary concept was considered to be more meaningful and
civilized than the scaffold or forms of corporal punishment that
were commonly used at that time. In the second, the city government derived economic advantage from it.

The institution had in 1599 already acquired a monopoly on the
rasping of wood for the ship-building industry. Having this hard and
unpleasant work done by prisoners cut two ways. First, the earnings
enabled the house of detention to be run without financial aid from

the city government. Second, it was reasoned, the prisoners, who were recruited from the ranks of vagabonds and other socially useless and dangerous idlers, through hard labour (sometimes fourteen hours a day) could be reformed into hard-working members of society who, after their release, would be able to earn an honest living.

In the seventeenth century the countless visitors to the rasping house from England, France, Scandinavia, Hungary, Italy and Germany took home enthusiastic reports. This enthusiasm was not always based on the humanitarian starting-points of Coornhert and Spieghel. In his study, *The Embarrassment of Riches, an Interpretation of Dutch Culture in the Golden Age*, Simon Schama relates that many of these foreign visitors actually 'were struck by the formidable system of disciplinary punishments that backed up the house regime' (Schama 1987: 23). This was another factor to which the Dutch prison system owed its fame. The system varied from deprivation of meat rations to floggings at the post with a 'bull's pistle'.

The reputation of the Dutch prison system was also partly based on fiction and hearsay. The most persistent fiction is that of the water cell, mentioned in many reports. Inmates of the rasping house who refused to work were said to be moved to more industry by a treatment in this cell. The earliest description of this dates from 1612:

> In the vestibule or entrance to the house there is running water, and beside it, a room with two pumps one on the outside and the other in the inside. The patient was brought thither so that by pumping into the room first as high as his knees, then as high as his waist, and as he was not yet prepared to give his attention to St. Pono [that is, to the devotion to labour] as high as his armpits, and finally up to his neck, when fearing he would drown, he began his devotion to St. Pono by furious pumping until he had emptied the room, when he discovered that his weakness had left him and he had to confess his cure. (Schama 1987: 23)[3]

Schama points out that this sole and – apparently – authentic Dutch source was actually a satirical pamphlet to which little or no realistic content could be ascribed. The title of the pamphlet, *History of the Wonderful Miracles . . . in a place called the tuchthuis*, also suggests rather 'a bizarre fable' or 'a sadistic fantasy, concocted from half-digested gobbets of hearsay' (Schama 1987: 23). Nevertheless, for two centuries the reputation of the 'progressive' Dutch penitentiary system was inseparably tied to the highly praised water cell and other disciplinary punishments.

### 1777: the isolation cell

It is to John Howard's credit that he did not allow himself to be misled by rumours, but based his description of the foreign penitentiary systems, in *The State of the Prisons*, rather on level-headed personal observation. He made short work of the water cell: 'On careful inquiry, I learned, that what has been said of a cellar, in which such transgressors are put to pump or drown, is not fact' (Howard 1977: 126). This, however did not lessen John Howard's admiration for the Dutch prison system. He applied different measures, such as: differentiation in execution of punishment (separate prisons for men, women, juveniles and the mentally disturbed); the mildness of the criminal law (the relatively limited use of imprisonment, the possibility of early release, the relatively short term of imprisonment); the quality of medical and mental care; hygienic conditions within the prison; and the use of paid labour as a means of correction. These characteristics made a strong impression on Howard. Their aim, just as it had been two hundred years earlier, was correction and reform. In contrast to the days of the rasping house, prison sentences were undergone in complete isolation instead of in small work-groups. The fiction of the water cell was replaced by the reality of the isolation cell in which the prisoner was kept day and night. This was done to prevent criminal infection and stigmatization and to increase the chance of moral and social improvement. These were the attributes which gave the Dutch prison system at the time of Howard its reputation of progressiveness, a reputation which it still enjoys today. But the question remains: how much of that reputation conforms with reality?

### 1989: the container cell

Abroad, The Netherlands still has the reputation as a country with a mild penal climate. In this regard, reference is made, among other things, to the small number of prisoners per hundred thousand inhabitants and the relatively short term of the unconditional prison sentences. (See Table 5.1.)

90

*Table 5.1* Number of prisoners per 100,000 population on
1 February 1988

| | |
|---|---|
| Luxembourg | 103.4 |
| England and Wales | 96.6 |
| Austria | 96 |
| France | 92 |
| Turkey | 90.2 |
| Federal Republic of Germany | 86.7 |
| Portugal | 84 |
| Belgium | 70.5 |
| Denmark | 69 |
| Italy | 62 |
| Sweden | 61 |
| Norway | 47 |
| Netherlands | 36 |

*Source: Prison Bulletin* 10, December 1988: 20

However, it is risky to use, as so often is done, the average prison population as a criterion for the mildness of the penal climate, because such an approach does not take into account the extent of criminality, the types of crimes, or the relative length of prison sentences. This is especially relevant to the Dutch situation. A comparison of Dutch prison statistics with those of the neighbouring countries shows that a considerably higher percentage of Dutch prisoners receive a prison sentence that has to be served immediately. The average length of these unconditional prison sentences imposed by Dutch judges is, however, considerably shorter. In so far as the Dutch reputation derives from judicial sentencing policy, it is only in the short length of the unconditional prison sentence, not the frequency with which it is imposed: over 85 per cent of unconditional prison sentences in the past twenty years were shorter than six months, and more than half of these were of one month or less. Other factors that contributed significantly to this image of a liberal and humane penal climate were, among others, generous application of the so-called expediency principle by the Public Prosecutor (until recently, the prosecution of almost 50 per cent of all solved crimes was waived for policy reasons), the extensive network of public assistance through the Probation Service, and the manner in which prison sentences were executed.

This image has in recent years begun to deteriorate. This is due to the sharp rise in registered crimes that began in the 1970s in combination with the economic crisis of the same period, and which ultimately led to a complete deadlock in the penal system. The police could no longer carry out their responsibilities in the desired manner. The Public Prosecution Office and the judiciary were seriously overtaxed and the prison system had to contend with a shortage of cells. This shortage was largely due to a lack of good alternatives for short-term imprisonment on the one hand and the imposition of more and longer prison sentences on the other, mostly in connection with illegal drug trafficking. The concomitant increase in pre-trial detention, for which no adequate alternative exists, has also contributed to a continuing crisis in the prison system. These factors combined have led the government to publish a detailed policy plan, *Samenleving en Criminaliteit (Society and Criminality)* proposing a long-term solution to these problems by combating crime. The most important pillars upon which this plan rests are:

1 Reducing the number of short-term prison sentences by introducing alternatives that do not involve deprivation of liberty, such as the Community Service Order;
2 Combating the most common forms of petty crime, such as vandalism, shoplifting, and alcohol abuse, through a combination of official prevention measures with emphasis on restoring the function of social control and official supervision;
3 A tougher approach to the more serious forms of crime, which include not only those considered 'classical' serious crimes, but also the newer forms, such as large-scale bank and insurance fraud, practices with illegal corporations, serious environmental crime, as well as organized crime in the areas of drug traffic, illegal gambling, illegal arms traffic, white slavery, etc.

To bring this about, it has been suggested that the threat of punishment for a number of crimes be heightened, that new penal provisions be created, and that, together with an intensified tracing and prosecuting policy, prison capacity be considerably expanded. Realization of the latter is being pursued with such industry that in less than ten years prison capacity will be tripled.

The favourable reputation of the Dutch penal system is largely due to its starting-points and aims. While these – its tradition – have not been affected by the new policy plan, the same cannot be said of the process of implementation. There has been a tightening of the regime and the security measures within the prison (for example, mandatory urine tests for drugs and frisking), economizing on social, medical and psychological assistance, decreased facilities for sports and recreation, forced carrying out of prison sentences in institutions not meant for that purpose and the re-use of buildings which had earlier been written off – creating a discrepancy between reputation and reality. For a Dutch prisoner today, confinement in a container is not, in Schama's words, a 'bizarre fable or a sadistic fantasy' but an everyday reality, in spite of all the idealistic aims of the prison system.

## THE USE OF PRISON WITHIN THE DUTCH PENAL SYSTEM

With the introduction in 1886 of the Dutch Penal Code, the system of sanctions that had been borrowed from the French *code pénal* was greatly simplified. Besides imprisonment, the code recognized only two other main types of punishment: detention and fines. Prison was assumed to be the proper punishment for crime. Detention and fines were reserved for misdemeanours, or less serious offences. For certain crimes, a fine could in principle be imposed as an alternative punishment, but such a punishment was considered of an entirely different order and only suitable for the lightest form of the crime in question. More than a hundred years later, and without much change in the punishment status of crimes, the law now emphasizes that in principle the fine takes precedence over the prison sentence. The law now requires that in imposing a punishment or measure involving deprivation of liberty, the sentence must specify the reasons for choosing this type of punishment. In crimes for which prison is the statutory punishment, a fine may nevertheless be imposed. This represents official legal recognition of the primacy of the fine over the prison sentence.

The final step in the gradual reduction of imprisonment will be the introduction in 1990 of the Community Service Order as an independent fourth main type of punishment. This is meant as a replacement for a short prison term of up to six months. Practice has followed the legislator in this case. Every year about 5,000 prison sentences are replaced by Community Service; other criminal convictions, about three-quarters of the total, involve a fine. Detention as a main form of punishment is only incidentally used, mainly for notorious traffic offenders, and is in its implementation practically the same as the short prison term, so here we may forego a separate discussion of this type of sanction.

Another way in which the legislator has tried to limit the imposition of imprisonment is through the suspended sentence: the total lifting of punishment as long as certain conditions are kept. All prison sentences up to one year may be suspended. Since 1 January 1987 this opportunity has been extended to include prison sentences up to and including three years, with the restriction that at least two-thirds of the sentence must be served. In practice, the suspended sentence is second in frequency to the fine, in sentences imposed by the judge. Of all penalties imposed for crime, approximately a half are fines, more than a quarter are totally suspended sentences and somewhat less than one quarter are totally unconditional prison sentences. This means that in Dutch criminal law procedure, imprisonment still plays an important role, although it is no longer dominant.

A prison sentence can be determinate or can be for life. A sentence is at least for one day, and at most for fifteen years, or if the judge can choose between life imprisonment and a determinate sentence, at most twenty years. The minimum of one day applies to all punishable offences where a prison sentence can be imposed. The maximum varies according to the crime, but even with an accumulation of punishable offences they may not exceed the above mentioned fifteen or twenty years.

A convict sentenced to an unconditional prison term does not have to serve the entire term. At a certain time, usually after two-thirds of the sentence has been served, with a minimum of six months, the prisoner is eligible for early, supervised, release.[4] The original idea was that this supervised release be considered a privilege, a bonus for good behaviour during detention, and as a transitional phase between total deprivation of liberty and total freedom. For this reason, it was subject to conditions. In practice, the so-called 'conditional release' became a right of the prisoner with almost no control over his observance of the conditions. Since 1 January 1987 this right has been formally recognized by law, and the system of conditional release was replaced by unconditional automatic early release. Only in exceptional cases, for example when a prisoner has seriously misbehaved during detention, is it possible to encroach upon this right. Conditions can no longer be placed on automatic early release. Hence, revocation is no longer possible.

The relatively few long prison sentences have contributed to the high reputation of Dutch criminal procedure, but in recent years, there has been a turning of the tide. Alongside the gradual reduction of short prison terms can be found a marked increase in long prison terms and pre-trial detention. While the average prison term in 1982 lasted 3.2 months, in the subsequent six years it increased to 5.6 months (*Staatscourant* 1989). This is mainly due to the increase in serious crime, in particular to the enormous flood of drug cases.[5] The number of unconditional prison sentences for drug crimes makes up nearly 10 per cent of all unconditional prison sentences, while the total term imposed accounts for about 30 per cent of all sentences for Penal Code crimes.[6] In 1990 50 per cent of all prisoners are in some way connected with drug crime and almost a third of them are, or become, addicted during detention. In some prisons more than two-thirds of the prisoners are addicted to hard drugs.[7]

These figures will only increase when the plans for extending prison capacity are realized, for more than 60 per cent of this extra prison capacity is intended for drug offenders.[8] In 1981 the available prison capacity for adults was approximately 3,850 places. In 1989 there was a need for about 7,600 places. The estimate for 1994 is almost 9,000 places. This includes more than 600 places in institutions for mentally disturbed delinquents.[9] In 1990 about 6,000 male and female adult offenders are deprived of liberty in some way (offenders serving detention or prison sentences, pre-trial detention or detention at the government's pleasure).

This detention is being undergone in 33 remand centres, 26 prisons and 8 judicial and non-judicial institutions for mentally disturbed delinquents. These institutions have an average capacity of 100 cells. The smallest establishment houses 20 inmates and the largest about 150. Some penitentiary complexes include more than one institution. The so-called 'Bijlmerbajes' in Amsterdam, for example, consists of six high-rise apartment buildings, each containing a separate institution with its own administrator, staff, regime and supervisory commission.

A number of Dutch institutions date from the nineteenth century and can hardly satisfy present-day standards. Some of these have a wing structure, and others have Bentham's panopticon as a model. The establishments built in the last twenty years are in accommodation and facilities comparable to the living quarters built for students during the same period, except for the omnipresent electronic surveillance. Other institutions, in particular the open and semi-open ones, are housed in rebuilt barracks, in a former boarding house for migrant workers, in former monasteries and in an old mansion. The newest architectural design is a stack of containers, or prefabricated sections, placed in the yard of a prison or house of detention.

The average ratio of staff members to inmates in these institutions is 0.9:1; this includes everyone from the prison director to the organist and from the prison officers to the librarian and the psychologist. Together, the prison officers and workshop supervisors form about 60 per cent of the total staff.

## PRISON ORGANIZATION AND VARIETY

### Starting-points in the execution of prison sentences

The Dutch prison system is organized on a number of principles which together form a guide-line for the division into different types of prison, the spread of prisons throughout the country, the choice and training of personnel, and for the architectural structure of new institutions. These basic principles are set down in various national agreements, such as the Constitution, the Code of Criminal Procedure, the Penal Code, the Prison Principles Act, the Prison Decree-Law, and international agreements such as the European Convention for the Protection of Human Rights and Fundamental Freedoms, the International Covenant on Civil and Political Rights, and the European Prison Rules. The principles set down in these various forms of legislation provide the first line of ideas about the manner in which prisoners are divided among the different institutions, and influence the actual treatment of and relations with the prisoners. The most important starting-points are discussed below: the principle of minimal restrictions, the legal status of the prisoner, preparation for freedom, the community as a standard, differentiation and selection, and the centralization of penitentiary management.

### The principle of minimal restrictions

The Prison Principles Act stipulates that suspects who have not yet been convicted (that is, those in pre-trial detention) may be subject

96

to no restrictions other than those strictly necessary for their detention or to maintain order. A similar starting-point with no legal counterpart applies also to convicts. The government must concretely justify its encroachment on the civil rights of convicted prisoners and may not a priori assume itself justified. A prison sentence pronounced by the judge in principle can only imply the deprivation of physical liberty of a citizen, either as such (imprisonment), or for other reasons (pre-trial detention, detention at the government's pleasure, etc.). In concrete terms, this principle of minimal restrictions means that the prisoner has the same civil rights as any other citizen, unless the realization of these rights is impossible under the necessary conditions of detention. The prisoner has, for example, an active as well as passive right to vote, the right of association and assembly, the right of religious freedom, the right to marry, the right to freedom of expression and the right to privacy (for example, the right to consult his or her own doctor or specialist).

The notion that imprisonment only means physical deprivation of liberty, no more and no less, and that every element of harsher punishment must be avoided, is not entirely unchallenged. In the literature and on the political level it is regularly suggested that the mildness of the penitentiary system on this point has gone too far (Teldersstichting 1988: esp. 61ff.; van Veen 1986: 28–42). Particularly with regard to the perpetrators of serious crimes there is a plea for turning back the clock and for developing a special prison sentence where the principle of minimal restrictions would not apply. This category of prisoner should be subjected to a harsher regime involving, among other things, no extended visiting, strict visitation rules and separation of the prisoner from the visitor by a glass partition, restricted use of the telephone, much restraint in the granting of leave, and abolishment of the right to automatic early release. Up to now, the legislator has not followed this line of thinking.

## The legal status of the prisoner

It is inevitable that every judicial deprivation of liberty brings with it a lowering of the legal status of the citizen in custody. However, the question will always arise of which rights might be retained in prison and which must be given up. The central point is the legal protection of the citizen against the state. In the 1970s and 1980s, especially under the influence of the new Utrecht school, led by Peters and later by Kelk, the emphasis on the protective rather than the instrumental function of criminal law, significantly contributed to the reform of criminal procedure.[10]. This signally concerns the area of criminal law administration where until recently there was an almost complete lack of legal protection: the detention phase. Geurts has emphatically called attention to this matter (Geurts 1962). There was an almost total lack of any formal regulation of legal status. In so far as it was possible to talk about a material legal status, it was primarily based on favours, not on rights that could be demanded. Rights were granted solely by the prison authorities, who had broad discretionary powers both in this respect and in the imposition of disciplinary punishment. Supervision was almost completely absent, since the prisoners had no right of complaint or appeal. Deprivation of liberty leads not only to dependency and arbitrariness, but also to deprivation or limitation of a number of essential rights which in themselves had no relation to detention (right to vote, freedom of religion, privacy of correspondence, right to certain social payments).

Now, in the last decade of the century, the legal status of prisoners has been considerably improved: a legally guaranteed contestable complaint and appeal procedure has come into existence and disciplinary punishment has been considerably mitigated. Detention law has developed from a fairly neglected area of criminal law into a speciality, the influence of which on other areas of law cannot be underestimated. The law on 'strengthening the legal status of prisoners' (Prison Principles Act 1977) now enables a prisoner to lodge a complaint with the complaints commission of his institution against any disciplinary punishment imposed upon him,[11] as well as any measure imposed upon him by or through the director, which deviates from the rights granted him by the regulations of the institution. Explicitly mentioned is the violation of his right of correspondence and of visitation. The complaints commission is formed by three members of the Supervisory Commission. The latter is a mandatory board for all institutions, consisting of independent citizens, and including a judge, a lawyer, a doctor and a social work expert, whose job is to supervise 'the treatment of the prisoners in the institution and the observation of the regulations established in their regard'. The complaints commission can wholly or partly revise a decision made by or through the director if:

1   The decision is in conflict with a prison regulation;
2   The decision, after assessment of all pertinent interests and cir-
    cumstances, is considered unreasonable or unfair.[12]

In certain cases the prisoner may be awarded money or some other
form of compensation. Both the plaintiff-prisoner and the director
of the institution can appeal to a higher body in The Hague.

Apart from the fact that the complaint is not handled in public,
the complaint procedure is in all aspects covered by legal guarantees. It is a contestable procedure in which both sides are heard,
with the possibility of conducting a defence and hearing witnesses.
The prisoner-plaintiff has a right to free legal assistance and the
decision must be communicated in writing and accounted for to the
party involved.[13] Together with this advanced elaboration of the
prisoner's right of complaint – a development which according to
Kelk is unique in the world (Kelk 1983: 8) – the 1977 law involved a
number of alterations in the disciplinary punishments to be applied
within the institution. Among others, the following were abolished:
confinement in a punishment cell; putting in chains; provision of
only bread and water rations; withholding of visitation, of the right
of correspondence, of reading material, of canteen articles, etc. In
their place, new disciplinary measures were instituted: isolation in
the cell for a maximum of two weeks, a fine and a reprimand. Partly
in connection with these far-reaching revisions of the Prison Principles Act, the Prison Decree-Law was also improved in many of its
aspects. These include: allowing more extensive contacts outside the
institution (correspondence, telephone conversations, improvement in the way information is provided, including to non-Dutch-
speaking prisoners, abolition of mandatory prison uniforms and
broadening of the regulations for leave). The 1977 complaints and
appeal legislation has given rise to an extensive jurisprudence
which, in Kelk's words, can be characterized by 'refinement of
justice, further elaboration of norms and rules and filling gaps in the
regulations, in regard to both material and procedural norms in the
detention situation' (Kelk 1983: 8).

### The resocialization principle

Since 1951, the leading principle in the execution of prison sentences has been that 'while preserving the character of the punishment or measure, its execution should serve the preparation of the

prisoner for his return to society' (Prison Principles Act 1977, article 57). It has come under pressure in recent years because of economy measures and the filling of penitentiary institutions beyond their capacity. Nevertheless, preparation for return to society is still the main principle determining what happens inside the institution. It is realized in many ways, not so much in the sense of granting favours, but rather by offering facilities to which every prisoner is entitled.

Thus, every institution provides the opportunity for education and training, for social and religious counselling differentiated as much as possible according to the various beliefs, for courses in creative and social skills, for taking part in discussion groups and for the use of the library facilities. Specialized officials have been appointed to fulfil all these tasks. Together with the provision of these internal facilities, the attempt is made to hinder as little as possible contact with the outside world. In practice, this means that the prisoner has visiting rights (a minimum of one hour every fourteen days), the right to free correspondence with anyone (in a number of institutions without supervision of the director) and, depending on the regime, the right to make and receive telephone calls and to go out on leave. Although still considered a favour, various forms of leave have in recent years increasingly been granted.

In addition, prisoners are allowed to have radio and television in their cells. This is done not only to improve knowledge of the outside world but also to save on personnel costs. Video programmes are increasingly replacing active recreational facilities. The communal execution of the prison sentence, and the differentiation and selection to be discussed below, are also ways of putting into effect the resocialization principle.

## Community life as a standard

In Howard's time also, the resocialization principle played an important role in carrying out the prison sentence. Then, unlike now, it was thought that this could best be achieved through reflection in total isolation. In 1951, the legislator broke radically with the existing system of cells. The Fick Commission, which prepared these alterations, looking back at this cell system, wrote: 'One does not know which is more striking: the noble character of the writers, the integrity of their intentions, their admirable philanthropy, or their

100

truly frightening lack of any psychological insight.'[14] This does not mean that the legislator has completely abolished detention in a cell. The starting-point is now that the prisoner should spend most of his day in the company of others, and the remaining time, the time for a good night's rest, in the cell. In a number of institutions prisoners also receive their meals in their cells. This is viewed as part of the prisoner's right to privacy. Plans of the justice department to solve the cell shortage by putting more than one prisoner in a cell have therefore met with much opposition, largely from the prisoners themselves, and have subsequently been withdrawn.

## Differentiation and selection

Criminal contamination, which in Howard's time was combated by completely isolating each prisoner, is now avoided by internal and external differentiation. External differentiation means the designation of separate prisons for groups of prisoners who 'fit' together according to certain criteria. Internal differentiation and selection occur within the institution itself. Criteria for differentiation and selection are: sex, age, length of prison term and type of crime, personality, assumed degree of dangerousness, nationality and domicile of the convict. Another criterion is whether the convict was already in custody at the time of his sentencing. Nowadays it is also taken into account whether the prisoner is addicted to drugs or alcohol. Some of these criteria are stipulated by law, and others have developed in practice.

This means that prisons have developed into one type or another. There are prisons and houses of detention for women, men or juveniles, in open, half-open or closed institutions, institutions for short or for long prison terms, institutions for those who have 'turned themselves in' or those already in pre-trial detention, in special institutions for traffic offenders (drunken drivers), for the mentally disturbed, or for dangerous criminals.

In addition, for some years experiments with 'day detention' have been in progress (in effect, meaning return to prison each night), especially as a means of preparing the detained for the return to society, and with 'weekend imprisonment'. A series of the latter type is exclusively meant for short-term prisoners.

Together with external differentiation, internal differentiation also takes place, most clearly in the larger institutions. This means that within an institution special sections of wings are arranged

101

according to the needs of certain categories of prisoners, such as drug addicts, escape-prone or otherwise dangerous criminals, and mentally disturbed prisoners. More and more institutions are setting up special 'drug-free' sections for ex-drug addicts or for prisoners who do not wish to come in contact with drugs. These sections or wings are characterized by a different regime from that of the rest of the institution. The above mentioned selection and differentiation takes place at different times.

It is important to note that neither the judge who imposes the sentence nor the public prosecutor, though formally responsible for the implementation of the prison sentences, may interfere with the manner of execution. Selection and differentiation still remain the business of the administration; it runs four selection advice committees which must give advice in the selection of, respectively, juveniles and adults with short prison terms, long-term prisoners, and candidates for open institutions. The administrations of the prisons concerned also take part in these selection advice committees. Selection within the institutions takes place under supervision of the director, according to internal procedures.

## Centralized management

Since the beginning of the nineteenth century, prison management has become more and more centralized. This is true of the relations within the institution as well as the relations between the institution and the Department of Justice. Final authority over all prisons is in the hands of the Minister of Justice. He determines the domestic regulations of the various institutions as well as the limits within which the prison director must remain in carrying out his duties. The authority of the department over the individual institutions is further emphasized in a number of regulations. For instance, permission to interrupt a sentence or to leave an institution must be granted by the minister; he also regulates the diet of the prisoners. However, the all-powerful minister can sometimes be forced by law to make concessions. Moreover, the legal provisions in which certain powers of the minister are set down are rather 'openly' formulated. The minister can do almost anything, but does not have to do everything. In practice this means more autonomy for the prison director. This tendency has been quite noticeable in the last few years. Recently, directors have been able to establish their own personnel policy and to make independent decisions regarding shifts in the budget of the institution. Decision-making within the institution itself also seems to be overly centralized in the person of the director. According to the Prison Decree-Law, article 7, the officials who work in the institution must strictly obey the director. But even here his authority is not absolute. When charged with making certain decisions the director is obliged to seek advice. The advisory procedure is spelled out in the domestic regulations. In addition, these regulations require certain 'discussions' to be held, several examples of which will be mentioned below in the description of the Breda Remand Prison. Finally, the director can delegate certain duties to his subordinates without losing his final authority.

### Detention in practice

The organization of the Dutch prison system broadly outlined above can be seen as well thought-out, advanced and consistent. But it is not just the theoretical concept which is important here, but rather implementation in daily practice. In this respect the picture is less optimistic. This is not so much due to shortcomings of the concept itself, but rather to the cell shortage, the far-reaching economy measures and the concomitant hardening of the penitentiary and criminal law climate. This has increasingly led to the overshadowing of penitentiary practice by a return to repressive measures.

An important factor is also the change in prison population. We have already mentioned the sharp increase in unconditional, long prison sentences. While up till now the majority of prisoners were those serving short prison terms, there is now a tendency – in itself praiseworthy – to replace the short prison term of up to six months with alternatives not involving deprivation of liberty, in order that the existing and still to be realized prison capacity can be reserved for long prison sentences. This means that the composition of the prison population is subject to considerable change. Drug addicts, foreigners, mentally disturbed individuals and hardcore criminals now form its nucleus. Problems resulting from this are: the danger of contamination by AIDS, deterioration of relations among the prisoners (drug dealing, corruption, threats, use of violence), racial conflicts, anxiety among personnel and prisoners. Add to this the buildings, which very often are out of date, or the emergency facilities which have hastily been put together, the personnel shortage (not only quantitative but also qualitative), and the relative decrease in funds, and here is a fact of life for which the theoretical concept has no answer.

In this state of affairs the differentiation and resocialization principles are losing their meaning. The penitentiary authorities, headed by the Ministry of Justice, are looking for an answer to this problem, but increasingly less in accordance with the principles described above, and more in measures for supervision, security and repression. The atmosphere from day to day is determined by compulsory urine tests, increased supervision of visiting, body searches, diminishing recreational possibilities and restrictions in granting leave. All this leads to tension not only among the prisoners but also among the personnel, not to mention the tension between personnel and prisoners. Such a climate is not conducive to a humane and resocialization-oriented treatment. Under these circumstances the danger exists that even good prison rules and regulations, still one of the most important pillars on which the penitentiary concept is based, may not work or may even be counter-productive.

## THE BREDA REMAND PRISON

### Introduction

In the following section we describe one of the sixty-seven Dutch penitentiary institutions. For several reasons, we have chosen a remand prison. Most prisons are of this type and most prisoners are detained in such an institution. Pre-trial custody alone accounts for almost 40 per cent of the entire Dutch prison population.[15] Despite what the name suggests, a remand prison is not only used for pre-trial detention, but also, because of the cell shortage, for short and medium sentences. The remand prison also functions as a prison for fine-defaulters, as a temporary holding place for deported foreigners and as an intermediate station for long-term prisoners and mentally disturbed delinquents waiting to be placed in a long-term prison or psychiatric institution. The remand prison therefore has a more heterogeneous population and presents a more representative picture than a specialized prison. In addition, the Breda Remand Prison is one well known to one of the authors, a member of the supervisory board.

The Breda Remand Prison is intended mainly for male prisoners. It has a capacity of 107 places, 8 of which are intended for temporary

104

detention. The remaining 99 places are primarily intended for those in pre-trial detention and those sentenced to prison. In addition there are four so-called 'isolation cells' for undergoing disciplinary punishment in the form of solitary confinement. (Solitary confinement may not exceed 14 days.)

The Remand Prison is a closed institution which means, among other things, that security plays an important role. Within the limits of optimal security, and with the restrictions deriving from the arrangement of the building, the institution endeavours to achieve the following objectives:

1 A humane execution of the detention;
2 The prevention or limitation, as much as is possible, of the damaging effects of detention;
3 The provision of individual assistance in building up the prisoner's resilience for when he returns to society.

Later we will see what these objectives actually mean with regard to how things work in the institution. But, in the next two sections we will first take a closer look at the Breda Remand Prison's building and the security measures. Some years after completion of the dome-prison, or panopticon, in Breda, work was begun at the rear on a new court-house and a house of detention. This came into use in 1892. The Prison Principles Act of 1951 designated it both as a house of detention for men and women and as a government workhouse for women. This last designation was short-lived, as less than a year later its function was taken over by the house of detention in Middelburg. Since the women's section was closed in 1960 it had one function, as a house of detention for men. This changed again on 1 January 1990, when it reverted to offering facilities for both men and women.

Because of the increasing need for special prisons for women the house of detention was then reserved for women. The men's house of detention was moved to the container cells (k) and to the adjacent panopticon (j). The building has been modernized several times over the years. In the 1970s, a new three-storey administration building was built, with room on the ground floor for the reception, administration and management (c). On the second storey there are a room for staff members, a library, an education centre and a recreation hall, while on the top floor the staff members' rooms and

105

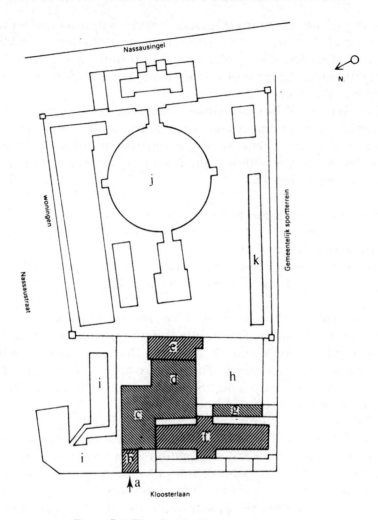

*Figure 5.1* The Breda Remand Prison

Key:
(a)  Entrance
(b)  Front part of the building
(c)  Director's office; administration; On the second storey: sport/recreation hall
(d)  Work-rooms
(e)  Gymnasium
(f)  Prisoners' living quarters
(g)  Punishment/isolation section
(h)  Exercise yard
(i)  Former court-house
(j)  Panopticon (special prison, the 'Boschpoort')
(k)  Container cells

*Source:* Adapted from Jonkers, W.H.A., *et al.* (1979) *Het penitentiar recht (Penitentiary law)* 10: 311

a hall for religious services are situated. To the left of the administration building on the ground floor are the isolation cells (g) and to the right the yard for exercising the prisoners (h). At the back are the work-rooms (d) and the gymnasium (e). Next to the administration block is the prisoners' living quarters: a rectangular block of cells, with two wings on the upper floors (f).

The standard facilities in each cell include a bed, a table and chair, a night table, a clothes closet and an armchair. Ninety per cent of the cells have a television set; they are rented for 6.70 florins a week ($3).

In 1984 it had been established that the building could no longer meet present-day standards. There were no toilets or running water in the cells, the washing and shower facilities were in a deplorable state and security could no longer be satisfactorily guaranteed. There was a general lack of maintenance throughout, which necessitated far-reaching renovation. This has been carried out in stages since 1986 and was completed in 1989 by the installing of a toilet and washing facilities in every cell. It is remarkable that the institution has been able to remain in use during this building period. This was only made possible by a great extra effort on the part of the personnel to keep security, reception and counselling at an acceptable level, and by adjustments in the institutional regime.

*Security*

Security has been considerably improved as a result of the above mentioned renovation. There has been an effort at eliminating the flaws in the security system and, among other things, the following have been put into use:

1  A new, protected entrance area (a), with a waiting room for visitors; it is equipped with a detection-gate;
2  A new visiting hall for visitors and new consulting rooms for legal counsel, rehabilitation, etc., the use of which prevents much of the movement of prisoners and visitors in and through the entire institution;
3  Observation by camera along the wall of the yard where prisoners take exercise, a measure which further improves security;

4 An automatic call-up and alarm system for the security personnel, to safeguard those who are regularly alone with groups of prisoners. The nature of the prison population is changing and staff have been in more personal danger in recent years. Security measures therefore taken include: regular cell inspection; detection routines for visitors and prisoners; frisking and inspection of body and clothing of prisoners. The system is now completely operational.

## The prison population

To give a picture of the average prison population in Breda, we will describe the situation on 1 April 1988 (Ministry of Justice 1988 1, 2). On that day there were 107 inmates. The average prison term of 165 days was well above the national average of 130 days.

Of the 107 inmates, 67 per cent were in remand or pre-trial detention, 7 per cent were under 'subsidiary' detention, 24 per cent were serving prison sentences and 2 per cent were waiting for a place in an institution for mentally disturbed delinquents. The crimes for which they were imprisoned were: larceny and embezzlement 42 per cent, violent crimes 22 per cent, drug crimes 19 per cent, sexual offences 7 per cent, misdemeanours 5 per cent, and various other offences 5 per cent.

Personal characteristics of the prisoners were as follows. Almost 30 per cent were 23 years of age or younger, 36 per cent were between 23 and 30, 20 per cent between 30 and 40, and 14 per cent were older than 40. Eighty-two of the prisoners were Dutch, 10 were Turkish, 11 were Moroccan, and 4 had other nationalities. This variation in nationality is reflected by the religious beliefs. Slightly more than 21 per cent were Islamic, about 48 per cent Roman Catholic, about 9 per cent Protestant, and 3 per cent professed another religion. Regarding the addiction problem, the picture coincides fairly well with the national picture in prisons: 21 per cent were addicted to hard drugs, and 9 per cent to alcohol. The same can be said for the level of education. On the average this did not go further than basic secondary school, plus, in most cases, an unfinished vocational training. An estimated 25 per cent of the prisoners were totally or partly illiterate.

## BREDA PRISON, HOLLAND

### *Treatment of the prisoners*

**The regime**

A humane treatment, aimed at limiting the damaging effects of detention and emphasizing individual assistance alongside security, is the basis for the regime. We will now take a close look at how this ideal is realized.

In the first place the prisoners at Breda should be suitably received, cared for and counselled. At first sight, the arrangement of the building does not lend itself to such an individually-oriented approach. The prisoners are housed in a cell building of three storeys. There is an open connection between the upper floors, allowing open and direct communication between them, and there are short walkways. The choice of an identical regime for all prisoners was partly due to this building arrangement and partly in order to maximize capacity. The disadvantages are that the prisoner may very quickly feel lost in the totality of the institution and that there is little room for personal contact between guards and prisoners.

Another objection is that no special facilities can be provided for the large group of alcohol and drug addicts, or for the mentally disturbed. The latter are being found more often in remand prisons as a result of capacity shortages in specialized mental institutions. The possibility for treatment for them within the remand prison is practically nil. The absence of a differentiated regime causes much tension in connection with the drug-related power structure, corruption of prisoners and supervisory measures on the part of the prison management (urine tests, cell inspection, visitation) which do not only affect addicted prisoners. The fear of the spreading of the AIDS virus among prisoners and personnel has recently arisen as a new problem. It is handled pragmatically, among other things by giving direct information within the institution and by handing out condoms to prisoners who request them. Since there has been no final decision on the national level about this problem, the prison management does not make syringes available to addicts. A compulsory AIDS test has been rejected in The Netherlands for ethical reasons.

In order to keep the negative effects of the uniform regime to a minimum, the prisoners have been divided among six living sectors. The prisoners in each are exercised together, participate jointly in the various activities, etc., and there is a permanent team of prison officers caring for and counselling them. The general rules governing the prison regime allow the prison management considerable freedom in putting the basic principles into practice, so the regimes of the various institutions vary considerably. The regime in Breda can be considered moderate. This is evident from the small number of complaints and appeals that have been lodged against management decisions, the flexible application of visiting and telephone regulations and the say allowed the prisoners by the management in matters concerning their own living situation.

## Personnel

Approximately sixty prison officers have a central role in the treatment of prisoners. Since 1977, the majority of prison personnel are no longer guards in the traditional sense, but officers who in addition to a security function also have the job of caring for and counselling the prisoners. At present prison officers share the responsibility for the treatment and counselling of prisoners and are very much involved in making recommendations about them. They are also expected to run activity programmes in the areas of recreation, sport, education and social and personal development completely on their own. This has had far-reaching effects on the quality of people sought for the position of officer.

While earlier a secondary school education was considered sufficient, supplemented by a short period of internal training, an increasingly specialized professional training is now required. Much attention is given to work counselling and in-service training. Nevertheless, many prison officers find the combination of security and counselling difficult. It is thus not surprising that the rate of absence due to illness is very high among prison officers; in 1987 it amounted to 14 per cent of the total work time. However, the character of most officers shows that resocialization is no empty promise.

In addition to the 60 prison officers there are 45 functionaries associated with the institution, 10 on a part-time basis. Besides management, administration and the 5 guards in the traditional sense (a total of 21 persons), we find among the functionaries: 3 religious counsellors, a doctor, a psychologist, a work counsellor, a social worker, 2 nurses, 2 organists, a teacher, a sports instructor, a librarian, 7 work superintendents, a bath superintendent, a canteen manager and a seamstress. Outside experts are also involved, such as: the district psychiatrist, the Islamic imam, the consultation bureau for alcohol and drugs, rehabilitation services, and the bureau of legal assistance. This last bureau holds a legal counselling hour for prisoners once a week in the prison.

The staff to prisoner ratio of 1:1 coincides with the national average. It is the most important expenditure in the prison system.The total cost of operating one prison cell per day, excluding personnel costs, is about 170 florins (about $80); including personnel costs, it comes to about 400 florins (about $190).

## Activities

The prisoners in Breda are able to take part in a broad range of activities. On the one hand this lessens the problem of idleness and boredom, and on the other the prisoner has to a certain extent the opportunity to plan his own day and thereby increase his self-sufficiency. This is also an attempt to check the process of de-personalization which is common in a total institution. For this reason too, the prisoners do not wear prison clothes, but are allowed to wear their own clothing. These are not to be considered favours, but rights to which the prisoner is entitled. This is especially true of activities that can be considered to be derived from their constitutional rights, such as the right to education, freedom of religion and freedom of association and assembly. At the same time, however, the prisoner who has chosen a certain activity is expected fully to participate in it and to do so with motivation.

The prescribed planning of the day enables as many prisoners as possible to take part in the programmes on offer. The day is divided into blocks, each with its own available facilities of which certain living-groups may make use. Some living-groups work during the morning block and have their recreational activities in the afternoon, while other groups have the reverse schedule. The activities in question can be divided into: labour or work, sports and fitness, education and library, arts and crafts, and group work led by the probation service. The idea that work has an important function in the resocialization process has remained unchanged since the days of the rasping and spinning houses. It is compulsory for prisoners. Non-prisoners, those on remand, also have a right to work.

In practice, more than 90 per cent of all inmates in Breda take part in work. Those who do not remain locked in their cells during work time. With the exception of weekends, the prisoners work a little over three hours a day. The work is done in five work-rooms and consists of the manufacture of fish boxes, packing and assembly work, metal work and textile work. It allows the prisoners to earn a maximum of 27.25 florins (about $13) a week.

Forty-five to 60 per cent of prisoners regularly take part in physical exercise and fitness-training lessons. At a fixed time the prisoners are called up in large or small groups to take part in various forms of exercise which are organized in a completely furnished sports hall, a fitness area and in the outside accommodation. There is an ample selection of sport activities: games such as football, hockey, volley-ball, basketball, badminton, and also fitness training, gymnastics and athletics. The prisoner may participate in these activities a minimum of twice and a maximum of four times a week.

Much attention is given to education. The teaching staff give courses in remedial education, literacy and social training. There are one Dutch and three foreign language courses, courses in secondary school subjects and in traffic education. In the education annex of the library, which was completely renovated in 1987, there is also a language laboratory. Efforts in education, however, are frustrated by the relatively short stay of prisoners in the institution and the resultant lack of continuity. In 1984 two small rooms were designated for arts and crafts, one for drawing and painting and the other for woodworking. The prisoners can participate once or twice a week in these activities; a maximum of six prisoners may at the same time be in one room. The probation service in the court district of Breda conducts group work with the purpose of helping people to meet one another, to exchange experiences and to help both one another and themselves. The groups are centred around a certain theme, such as addiction, justice and detention and the relationships of prisoners.

*Daily routine*

As an example of an average day in the prisoner's life in the Breda Remand Prison, we have chosen a Monday schedule:

| 06.55 | Morning call |
| 07.00 | Opening of the cells and roll call |
| 07.00–07.30 | Toilet and washing-rounds of 10 minutes per inmate, distribution of medicine, breakfast |

112

| | |
|---|---|
| 07.30–0800 | Planning the day |
| 07.45 | Bell for the morning work team |
| 07.50–11.00 | Work |
| 10.00–10.15 | Coffee break |
| 11.00–12.00 | Exercise outside of containers, cell inspection |
| 11.30 | Distribution of mail |
| 12.00–12.45 | Dinner in the cell |
| 13.00–14.15 | Library |
| 13.00–14.00 | Fitness |
| 13.00–14.30 | Arts and crafts |
| 14.15–17.00 | Opportunities for education (optional) |
| 14.15–15.45 | Visiting (twice a week for one hour) plus frisking and body search |
| 14.00–15.40 | Social consultation hour |
| 14.45–15.00 | Sports (max. 4 times a week) |
| 13.30–17.00 | Bathing on call (max. 4 times a week) |
| 15.15–15.30 | Tea break |
| 16.00–17.00 | Exercise |
| 17.45–18.30 | Supper |
| 18.45–21.30 | Recreation (max. 10 hours a week) |
| 19.00–21.15 | Discussion groups led by the religious counsellor |
| 19.00–21.45 | Opportunity to use the telephone (max. 10 minutes twice a week) |
| 20.15–21.15 | Toilet rounds |
| 21.45 | Locking in the cell |
| 23.00 | Lights out (or, on request, at 00.30) |
| 08.00–18.00 | Consultation with medical staff |

We have given a schedule for a group that works in the morning. The schedule for prisoners who work in the afternoon (from 13.30) is reversed.

Some facilities are available on other days than Mondays. The dentist has his consultation hours on Tuesdays from 8.30 to 14.00, discussion groups led by the probation service take place on Tuesdays, Wednesdays and Thursdays from 16.00 to 16.45, and the canteen is open on Thursdays from 8.00 to 12.00 and from 13.00 to 17.00. This is run by an outside grocer. The prisoners may spend up to 60 florins (about $25) a week on consumer goods. Payment is made via a current account system within the prison. Prisoners are not allowed to handle cash.

Apart from this schedule, a prisoner is allowed the opportunity on any day, though in principle not during work time, to be visited by his lawyer or rehabilitation officer, or to speak to an employee of the bureau of legal assistance. He may also ask to speak to members of the supervisory commission. One member of this commission, the so-called 'month-commissioner', visits the prison at least twice a month. He speaks to prisoners who have entered a request for this, and regularly attends meetings of the prisoners' committee. The month-commissioner also acquaints himself with other prison business, and is asked to visit every prisoner in solitary confinement. Every month he makes a report of his findings, a copy of which is sent to all members of the commission and the prison management, and which is discussed during the monthly commission meetings. Once a year the supervisory commission receives the entire prisoners' committee during such a meeting.

Every Saturday morning a barber is available in the prison. At weekends there is a simplified day schedule, without work, library, education or other training and sport activities. During the weekend the prisoner spends a lot of time in his or her cell, with only a church service, a few hours of recreation and the required exercise as variation. For the last few years, warm meals have not been prepared in the prison kitchen but have been delivered by a catering service. The prisoners have a wide choice on the menu. Dietary wishes for medical, religious or ideological reasons are taken into account. The schedule does not contain activities organized by the prisoners themselves. In the institution there is a prisoners' committee which, in consultation with the management, plans the programmes for public holidays and decides which video programmes are to be shown on the internal video network of the prison. Here special attention is paid to the wishes of foreign prisoners. The prisoners also publish their own magazine.

## Conclusion

Although the Remand Prison at Breda has not remained untouched by economy measures, shortage of capacity and the changing nature of the prison population, the climate has remained fairly moderate and individually-oriented. There is seldom serious tension among the prisoners themselves or between prisoners and guards. Many problems are solved informally. This relative stability is also evident from the number and types of official complaints made to the complaint commission of the supervisory commission. In relation to previous years the number of complaints has gone down considerably, as shown in Table 5.2.

*Table 5.2* Complaints made by prisoners at Breda Remand Prison

| Year | No. of complaints | No. of prisoners |
|------|-------------------|------------------|
| 1983 | 24 | 22 |
| 1984 | 30 | 22 |
| 1985 | 9 | 8 |
| 1986 | 46 | 20 |
| 1987 | 25 | 20 |
| 1988 | 6 | 6 |

The complaints were lodged in connection with disciplinary punishment for trying to escape (twice in 1988), exercise, food, censorship of an article for the prison magazine, and placement in solitary confinement because of danger of violence from other prisoners.

This has been a description of a typical prison in The Netherlands. There are prisons which are more open to the outside world, especially the open and half-open prisons; there are also those with a much stricter regime, namely the special prisons for those sentenced to long terms. There are prisons where the building arrangement is better, and there are also some which would suffer in comparison with Breda. Between these extremes the Breda Remand Prison, taking all aspects into account, gives a representative picture of the Dutch prison system. All things considered, this picture can still be called a positive one.

It is doubtful whether the same will be true after 1990, when the entire Remand Prison will be housed partly in the old, neighbouring panopticon and partly in the recently placed containers. Howard was one of the first to call attention to the influence of the buildings on the living climate in the prison. Two hundred years later, locking up prisoners in a panopticon and in containers shows that hardly any of this awareness remains.

## NOTES

1 For an overview of the history of the Dutch prison system and penal theory see: Hallema, A. (1958) *Geschiedenis van het Gevangeniswezen, hoofdzakelijk in Nederland,* The Hague, and de Monte-Verloren, J. Ph. (1937) *Geschiedenis der Nederlandse Strafrechtswetenschap,* Amsterdam.

2 A rasp was a coarse kind of file, used for scraping, rubbing down or finishing wood.

3 *Historie van de Wonderlijcke Mirakelen, die in menichte ghebeurt zijn, en de noch dagelijk ghebeuren, binnen de vermaerde Coop-stad Aemstelredam: In een plaats ghenaempt het Tucht-huys, gheleghen op de Heylighewegh* (1612), Amsterdam. The English translation of this fragment is by Simon Schama, in *The Embarrassment of Riches* (op.cit.), p.23.

4 Automatic early release, however, does not apply to those sentenced to life imprisonment. Such a prisoner can, via an appeal, ask that his sentence be commuted to a determinate one. He may then be released after serving two-thirds of his time.

5 See especially the departmental note *Samenleving en Criminaliteit, een beleidsplan voor de komende jaren (Society and Criminality, a policy for the coming year)* (1985), in which this issue is dealt with.

6 See Centraal Bureau voor do Statistiek (Dutch Central Statistical Office) (1987) *Criminaliteit en Strafrechtspleging (Criminality and Criminal Law Procedure)* and Interdepartementale Stuurgroep Alcohol-en Drugbeleid (ISAD) (Interdepartmental Steering Committee for Policy on Alcohol and Drugs) (1986) *Heroverweging 1986 Drug-en alcoholbeleid (Reconsideration 1986 of policy on drugs and alcohol),* annex 6, pp. 5–6.

7 See Interdepartementale Stuurgroep Alcohol-en Drugbeleid (ISAD) (1985) *Drugbeleid in beweging (Drug policy in motion),* p. 11; Erkelens, L.H. (1986) *Drugvrije detentie (Drugless detention),* The Hague: Government Advisory Group, p. 13; and the report (1985) *Drugvrije detentie (Drugless detention),* The Hague: Government Advisory Group.

8 See *Structuurplan Penitentiare Capaciteit (Master Plan Penitentiary Capacity)* (1985), The Hague: Justice Department.

9 These figures are based on the recent report *Voorzieningenbeleid delinquentenzorg en jeugdinrichtingen: 1990–1994 (Policy for facilities for delinquents and institutions for youth: 1990–1994)* (1989), The Hague: Justice Department, and on two reports *De capaciteitsprobelm bij het gevangeniswezen (Capacity problems in the prison system)* (June 1981), The Hague: Justice Department, and *De capaciteitsbenhoefte van het gevangeniswezen (Capacity needs of the prison system)* (January 1984), The Hague: Justice Department.

10 See among others Peters, A.A.G. (1972) *Het rechtskarakter van het strafrecht (The legal character of criminal law),* Deventer; Kelk, C. (1976) *Rapport rechtspositie gedetineerden (Report on the Legal Status of Prisoners),* Utrecht; *The Kempe-bundle: Recht-Macht-Manipulatie (Law-Power-Manipulation)* (1976) published by the Utrecht school, Utrecht; Kelk, C.

(1978) *Recht voor gedetineerden* (*Justice for Prisoners*), Alphen aan de Rijn; and *Kort begrip van het detentierecht* (*A short explanation of the detention law*) (1983), Nijmergen.

11 This commission was established by the Department of Justice on 5 November 1964. In 1967 the commission issued a final report which also contained a bill. A summary of the events that led to the change in the law and its further history was given by A.C. Guerts in his valedictory speech: 'De rechtspositie van de gevangene of hoe het was, is en zou kunnen zijn' ('The legal status of the prisoner: how it was, is and might be') Deventer, 1981.

12 Article 57, Beginselenwet Gevangeniswezen (Prison Principles Act).

13 For further information on the complaints and appeals law, see: Kelk, C. (1978) *Recht foor gedetineerden,* op.cit.; Balkema, J.P. (1979) *Klachtrecht voor gevangenen* (*Complaints law for prisoners*), Alphen aan de Rijn; Jonkers, W.H.A., *et al.* (1979) *Het penitentiar recht* (*Penitentiary law*), Arnhem; Van Ratingen, P. (1983) *Recht en gevangenschap* (*Law and imprisonment*), Deventer.

14 Report of the Commissie voor de verdere uitbouw van het Gevangeniswezen (Commission for the further development and extension of the prison system) (1947), Staatsdrukkerij, The Hague, p. 9.

15 On 1 February 1989 in The Netherlands there were 5,291 persons imprisoned. The percentage of unconvicted prisoners, which are almost always kept in houses of detention, was at that time 38.5 per cent. See *Prison Bulletin* 10, December 1988, p. 20.

# REFERENCES

Coornhert, D.V. (1587) *Boeven-tucht ofte Middelen tot mindering der schadelyke ledighghanghers* (*Scoundrel reform, or the means of reducing dangerous idlers*), first published in Amsterdam.

Geurts, A.C. (1962) *De rechtspositie van de gevangene* (*The legal status of the prisoner*), Assen.

Howard, J. (1977) *The State of the Prisons* (bicentennial edn, facsimile reprint of first edn of 1777), Abingdon.

Jonkers, W.H.A., *et al.* (1979) *Het penitentiar recht* (*Penitentiary Law*), Arnhem: Gouda Quent.

Kelk, C. (1983) *Recht voor Geinstitutionaliseerden* (*Justice for the Institutionalised*), Arnhem.

Ministry of Justice (1988) *Beleidsplan huis van bewaring Breda* (*Policy plan, Breda Remand Prison*), Breda, supplement 3.

Schama, S. (1987) *The Embarrassment of Riches, an Interpretation of Dutch Culture in the Golden Age,* London: Collins.

*Staatscourant,* government newspaper, 28 August 1989.

Teldersstichting, B.M. (1988) *Strafecht en rechtshandhaving* (*Criminal law and law and order*), The Hague: Liberal Party Working Group Report.

van Veen, Th.W. (1986) 'Wat beneemt de vrijheidsstraf?' ('What does prison take away?'), in *100 jaar vrijheidsstraf* (*100 years of imprisonment*), Groningen.

*Chapter Six*

# MATAGALPA PRISON, NICARAGUA

## *GINNY BAUMANN AND KEVIN BALES*

## INTRODUCTION

Nicaragua is a nation in transition, and its prison system reflects the remarkable and sweeping changes in life and government since the end of the Somoza dictatorship in 1979. These changes, such as the transfer of land to co-operatives and poorer peasants, the literacy campaign and the present drive to clean up the country's water sources, all demonstrate a thrust of government policy very different from the regime which ended in 1979. In many ways the Nicaraguan prison system is an exemplar of this shift in political philosophy and policy.

Many of the current members and officials of the Nicaraguan government were held in the nation's prisons prior to the revolution. A government with such a high proportion of its members having first-hand and intimate knowledge of prison life is rare, and explains, in part, the equally rare views of the Nicaraguan government on the nature of imprisonment. On the continuum of penal philosophy which stretches from the punitive to the reformative, the Nicaraguan penal system has placed itself on the far edge of reform.

The pursuit of these principles by the Nicaraguan penal system occurs within strict shortages of basic resources. Two political situations have detracted from the physical improvement of the prison system. The first of these and the most immediate was the war which was fought along the Honduran border and elsewhere between the Nicaraguan forces and the 'Contras', who were armed and supported by direct grants from the US Congress. Government resources have been constantly diminished by the need to prioritize defence.

In addition to the consumption of resources by the Contra war, it might well be expected that military invasion would harden government attitudes towards those whose actions were deemed anti-social or anti-government. It is certainly true that a State of Emergency was in effect for most of the period of hostilities, being lifted in January 1987. This State of Emergency restricted certain freedoms, including the right of habeas corpus (restored in non-political cases in 1985). However, the State of Emergency did not suspend other significant sections of the Statute of Rights and Guarantees of Nicaraguans. In particular those articles of the statute survive which forbid cruel, inhuman, or degrading punishment. The abolition of the death penalty following the revolution remained intact. As will be discussed below, the treatment of detainees suspected of security offences is still open to serious questioning, but the operations of the penal system itself continue within the bounds set by the Statute of Rights.

The second limiting factor was less immediate, but of greater potential impact. This was the trade embargo which was enforced on Nicaragua by the United States. Before the revolution the USA was, by far, Nicaragua's most important trading partner. Today the impact of the embargo is to be seen everywhere in the economy, as well as in the prisons. Despite the fact that the government has greater calls on its meagre resources than building more comfortable prisons, the physical plant of the prisons has been steadily improved. Workshops and gymnasiums, for example, have been added to the main prisons. Most prison facilities are now operating below their capacity and, unlike those in many more industrialized countries, do not suffer significantly from overcrowding. In Central America it stands out as a model of high quality provision drawn from a small resource base.

## THE PRISON SYSTEM

In 1980, just after the revolution, the Inter-American Commission on Human Rights visited Nicaragua and inspected ten prisons around the country. Seven of these ten they regarded as 'deplorable' – overcrowded, poorly serviced, and dilapidated. Their report explained these conditions in terms of the inheritance of the crumbling Somoza penal system. 'Of necessity', they wrote, 'the Government had to use the former regime's detention institutions, which in the best of times had been rudimentary and which deteriorated notably in the years prior to the fall of Somoza' (IACHR

1983: 99). Americas Watch also found crowded prisons in 1982, primarily in the two main prisons which were used to house 'Somocistas'. Since the inspection of the system in 1982 many changes have taken place, particularly in the physical plant and in the organization of the prison regime. In broad outline: the prison population of Nicaragua is estimated at a little over 7,000 inmates. About 235 of these are members of the Nicaraguan army or police serving sentences imposed by military courts. Of the remainder about three-quarters (5,328) are common-crime offenders. Another one-fifth (1,515) are either charged or convicted of security-related offences. This latter number had been much larger; it included, until the recent amnesty, more than 2,000 former National Guardsmen and others convicted by the 1979–81 special courts; of these only 39 remained in prison in October 1989.

There are two main prisons in Nicaragua, fifteen small prison farms, and a number of detention centres run by the Directorate General of State Security. The prison at Tipitapa, near Managua, is the largest. Until the recent amnesty it housed just under 3,000 inmates at 80 per cent capacity; some 2,000 of these were former members of the National Guard. The other major prison, Heroes y Martires de Nueva Guinea (or 'Zona Franca') is also near Managua, and is used for those awaiting trial. The fifteen prison farms, including one for women, are recently-built, low security facilities. In addition to the main prisons and prison farms there are gaols in several cities.

The prisons are classified as open, semi-open, or closed. The allocation of inmates to any one of these depends on their participation in the five-stage programme which leads to probation and release. The five stages are:

Stage 1: A closed ordinary prison system, without work;
Stage 2: A closed prison, but the inmate is allowed to work and receives privileges and more family visits. If an inmate demonstrates good behaviour he or she may, after serving 30 per cent of the sentence, progress to a semi-open system. Most inmates progress to this second stage immediately after conviction and sentencing, depending upon their willingness to join in work programmes and education;
Stage 3: A semi-open prison or low security gaol, the inmate being free to move about the grounds and working outside the

facility during the day. After serving a further 20 per cent of their sentence in a semi-open regime, inmates are moved on to an open system;

Stage 4: An open system with no security measures. Prison officials do not carry arms and the facility is run by an elected council of inmates. There are weekly visits, once a month the inmate is given a weekend leave, and once every six months is allowed home for a week. After another 10 per cent of the sentence is served in the open system of Stage 4, the prisoner is placed on probation and allowed to go home;

Stage 5: A probationary period in which the prisoner continues to report to the police, but lives and works normally. The prison officials are supposed to provide each probationer with employment at this stage in the rehabilitation process, but it is unclear whether or not this is possible in the current economic crisis.

As can be seen, the total sentence can be reduced by as much as 60 per cent if the prisoner is placed directly into Stage 2 after conviction. At all stages good behaviour and a good work record make possible the earning of more privileges. All prisoners are urged to pursue educational and cultural activities. Pardons and commutations are also granted on the basis of good behaviour, and there is a reasonable expectation of a sentence being reduced once a prisoner has progressed to the open system of Stage 4. As an example of the reduction of sentence, some inmates, including ex-National Guardsmen, serving twenty- to thirty-year sentences, had reached the open system of the fifth stage within eight years of incarceration. There has been one independent study of the open farm system (McCabe 1986). This study, conducted between 1982 and 1984, found a recidivism rate of 15 per cent among participants. It also stated that '90 per cent of the respondents indicated that their experience in the programme had helped them to see more clearly the forces at work in their lives and had in fact helped them to take more control over their lives'.

The International Committee of the Red Cross (ICRC) has made extensive and unrestricted visits since 1985, three or four times per year, to Tipitapa and Zona Franca. The Red Cross primarily visits those inmates who are former National Guardsmen or who have been sentenced for counter-revolutionary activity. In addition, since 1985, the Red Cross has run seminars, with government agreement, for members of the National Penitentiary Programme and the police.

Despite some criticisms which will be considered below, the basic assessment of the Nicaraguan Prison System must be positive. The Catholic Institute for International Relations, who inspected the system in 1986, stated that

> In a continent notorious for appalling prison conditions, where brutality and corruption are the norm, Nicaragua's penal system stands out as a genuine effort to find a more humane yet afford-able alternative. Such criticism as there is concentrates on lack of resources, which is a feature of the Nicaraguan economy as a whole and is not limited to the prison system. (1987: 66)

The Nicaraguan penal system has several features unique in Central America and, in the case of Matagalpa Prison, these special features are examined in more detail.

## MATAGALPA PRISON

The prison in Matagalpa had been built to hold a maximum of 600, and in January 1989 there were 530 occupants. Food consisted of a relentless but sufficient diet of rice and beans (typical of the population in general). Most of the prison seemed to be laid out in large open 'wards' with bunk beds rather than individual cells. There was a high standard of cleanliness throughout the prison. By the standards of some prisons in economically developed countries, Matagalpa prison was spartan and comfortless, but conditions seemed no worse than those faced by most of the rural population in Nicaragua.

Underlying the programme at Matagalpa is the belief that people are able to change in fundamental ways. The analysis of crime put forward by the present Nicaraguan leadership is one based mainly on social deprivation, lack of opportunities and corruption by values of greed and individualism. The Education Officer of Matagalpa Prison went as far as to say that when systems of exploitation can be brought to an end, crime as a major social phenomenon will disappear. This philosophy is matched by the general willingness of the Nicaraguan people to accept ex-offenders back into the community. It may be concluded that without the experience of events since

1979, this 'faith in the possibility of change' could not have become the guiding principle of the prisons.

If the aim of the prison system is to reform the individual, the method is education. This understanding of the role of education can partly be explained by the experience of the literacy campaign which was carried out throughout Nicaragua shortly after the revolution. This massive mobilization against illiteracy, mainly put into effect by older schoolchildren, brought basic reading and writing skills to all but 12 per cent of the population. Only months before this campaign, over half of the population were illiterate. The Nicaraguan government explains that this immediate involvement of the rural population and the huge changes and challenges which literacy brought to their lives is one of the main reasons that the revolution has been sustained.

In the prisons, formal education is available in the subjects taught in Nicaraguan schools, so that prisoners can complete the six grades of elementary schooling. It is worth stressing that all of this teaching is done by the prisoners themselves rather than by prison officers. Likewise any prisoner with skills in a basic trade will be encouraged to share them with other inmates. In the prison at Matagalpa, prisoners spoken with there seemed proud of the responsibilities they held as teachers and trainers in the prison. Prisoners being trained in woodwork explained that their major frustration was with the shortage of tools and materials.

Prisoners' education is enhanced by a wide range of cultural activities. The performance of dance and drama attended during the inspection of Matagalpa Prison was a good testimony to the efforts being made to draw out the creativity and self-expression of the prisoner. Inmates had the chance to join special groups for music, drama, dance and art. Complaints were of insufficient guitar strings, paints and brushes. Until the United States sanctions on Nicaragua and its backing for the Contra war come to an end, these limitations on living standards will continue to affect prisoners as much as they affect the rest of the population.

The education programme is an essential part of the five-stage progression through the prison system. The prisoners' willingness to participate in cultural, training and education activities is partly what determines the speed with which they move through the system and the frequency of access to various benefits. Equally important in deciding their progress is their willingness to join in work schemes.

At the bottom end of the ladder are those inmates, mostly Somo-cistas and ex-National Guardsmen, who refuse to work or join in education. They end up simply serving out the full term of their sentence, unless affected by the various amnesties. For those prisoners who co-operate, the regime is semi-open after the first third of their sentence. This means they are taken on a daily basis to farms and other work-places outside the prison. Prisoners are later transferred to open farm prisons. Each of these farms has only about fifty inmates, under very light surveillance by unarmed staff. Prisoners have a full-day visit from their families once a week. Those in open prisons have a 48-hour pass each month to go home, and have eight days 'holiday' twice a year. Last year, only 2 per cent broke the rules and disappeared. This frequent contact with families is given strong emphasis by the prison authorities, who see it as one of the key elements both of encouraging prisoners to participate and in preparing them for successful reintegration. Even as early as the second stage of imprisonment conjugal visits are permitted every fifteen days.

There is an attempt to involve the families in improving life in prisons and there are 'Family Councils' attached to each prison with the right to make proposals on education programmes, living con-ditions and on ways to resolve problems within prisons.

It is hard to be accurate about the 'success' of the Nicaraguan prison system in reforming offenders and reintegrating them into society. The government claims its success is shown by a remarkably low 5 per cent rate of recidivism.

## THE RIGHTS OF PRISONERS IN NICARAGUA

Part of Nicaragua's claim to be a 'freer' society lies in its treatment of offenders. Given the challenge to this claim by those who label the country 'totalitarian', the state of the prisons takes on a special significance. It is as true for Nicaragua as for any country that the full political importance of its prison system lies in its possible role as an instrument of social terror. The best way to illustrate this point is to show the role of prisons in the pre-revolutionary Nicaraguan regime.

Somoza's gaols were a central component of a huge apparatus of fear. They were, and were intended to be, a massive deterrent to political opposition. Under Somoza, there were scarcely any official prisons as such; rather, the National Guard command posts were used for detention. Reports from human rights organizations at the time indicate systematic abuse of prisoners, especially of political prisoners. The pervasive nature of torture, disappearance and killings and the fact that they went unpunished suggests that these violations were officially sanctioned. Men and women were not held separately and women in detention faced rape and physical abuse. A Matagalpa prison official claimed that the US government arranged for officials who had served in the Korean and Vietnam wars to go to Nicaragua to teach the National Guard methods of torture. Advisers came from Argentina for the same purpose.

The Nicaraguan government states that it has made a clear break with the use of imprisonment as a means of political repression. Chapter 1, Article 4 of the 1985 Ministry of Interior guide-lines sets out that the penitentiary system must completely end all types of torture, violence, physical or psychological mistreatment of prisoners. All prisoners are made aware of these rights.

At the head of the prison system is Tomas Borge, the Minister of the Interior. Just before the revolution he spent seven months in detention chained to a wall. At this time, his wife Yelva was tortured to death. Many of the present officials of the Nicaraguan government have their own horrific experiences to relate about Somoza's prisons. After these experiences they set out to rebuild the prison system, from the perspective of prisoners turned gaolers.

After the marking of Nicaragua's 'Tenth Year of Freedom' in 1989, how do the prisons measure up to the government's claims? The Nicaraguan government does not suggest that *all* abuses of prisoners have been overcome. As in any prison system, violations still occur. What it does claim, and what there is evidence for, is that anyone, of whatever rank, who uses violence or brutality against prisoners will be tried and punished if convicted. The Inter-American Commission on Human Rights reported that any prison warders found guilty of beating prisoners were punished. In the two principal Nicaraguan prisons, Tipitapa and Zona Franca, Americas Watch in 1982 'encountered no credible reports of beatings or similar mistreatment' (1984).

126

# TREATMENT OF FORMER NATIONAL GUARD MEMBERS

If any section of the Nicaraguan prison population were at risk, it would be those prisoners who had served in Somoza's National Guard. It is clear that the main prisons in which they are held are no longer overcrowded and that if they choose to do so, these prisoners can participate in the full range of activities. Until recently the most serious problem noted by outside observers was the approximately 1,000 former members of the National Guard who were held in Tipitapa and who refused to take part in the five-stage programme of rehabilitation. With a sizeable number of these prisoners now pardoned, this situation has apparently been resolved.

As well as those prisoners given an amnesty, the Catholic Institute for International Relations estimates that at least 260 ex-Somocistas have already worked their way through the five stages of imprisonment and, although given long sentences, have now been released on the basis of their behaviour. In 1989 most of the former National Guardsmen were released by the Nicaraguan government. This amnesty was part of an agreement made by Nicaragua with four other Central American countries in an effort to bring peace to the region. In March 1989 some 1,900 of these Somocistas were pardoned. Previously, in November 1987, 985 prisoners had been released.

The Nicaraguan government has found this policy of amnesty hard to make acceptable to the general public. Memories of National Guard atrocities are fresh in the popular mind; in the last year of the dictatorship between 40,000 and 60,000 people died at their hands. At the time of the pardon the Minister of the Interior, Tomas Borge, met many groups of the war-wounded and the relatives of past victims. In a speech made to one group he argued that they had need to 'give up some of [their] justifiable rage' (*Independent* 1989). On the same day President Ortega addressed a gathering that included women who held pictures of relatives killed by the Contras. In his address he stated that 'he wouldn't be in favour of the pardon, but peace is worth much more' (*Independent* 1989).

## PRE-TRIAL DETENTION

While there is sufficient evidence of protection of prisoners within the prison system itself, questions must be raised about the use of pre-trial detention. Under the State of Emergency, the Directorate General of State Security (DGSE) was allowed to hold people suspected of political offences indefinitely in detention for investigation. Serving inmates are also sometimes removed to these centres when they are suspected of involvement in other crimes. In some cases that were drawn to the attention of the Juridical and Human Rights Commission of the main Protestant organization (CEPAD), people had been held for as long as three months without being interrogated. Americas Watch estimated in 1986 that at any one time, 300 or more prisoners were held in DGSE facilities. This tallies fairly well with government figures.

It is disturbing that until recently there was no access to DGSE holding centres by Red Cross officials. But at the same time lawyers and family were generally permitted to make regular visits. Americas Watch stated that 'As best we can determine, torture as that term is generally understood is not practised in Nicaragua as a means of eliciting information or confessions, nor as a form of punishment' (Americas Watch 1984) but its report goes on to detail cases where harsh interrogation techniques were used (see also Amnesty International 1982). Americas Watch gives as examples prisoners put several days in small darkened cells, and the use of sleep deprivation and threats. Those testifying to these abuses often explained that their treatment was due to the intrigues of local government officials, who were accusing them of collaboration with the Contras. Talks between the government and opposition parties in the summer and autumn of 1989 led to improvements in the detention centres. Inspections were carried out by outside groups for the first time, and changes, such as putting windows into dark cells, took place.

## INVESTING IN BETTER PRISONS

It is a commonly understood element of the rights of prisoners that prison conditions should be such as to maintain life and health. It was particularly on the grounds of overcrowding and poor physical conditions that Nicaraguan prisons were severely criticized in the opening months of the new government.

In 1979, when it came to power after a long and vicious civil war the new government detained between 7,000 and 8,000 former members of the National Guard. Of these, 4,300 were tried and received prison sentences, and the rest were released. There was nowhere to put these prisoners except back into the former regime's gaols, where they did indeed face sub-human conditions, especially of overcrowding. In October 1980, the Inter-American Commission on Human Rights reported on this situation. By the time the report was published, three out of ten of the inspected prisons had already been shut down. Americas Watch said that by 1986 overcrowding had been solved in the largest prison (Tipitapa), and inmates had more facilities for work and recreation and for family visits. As explained above fifteen new 'open farm' prisons have been constructed and more of these are essential if the Sandinista prison guide-lines are to be fully put into action.

In Matagalpa, the achievements of the prison system were reflected in the very positive attitude of inmates and in the aspirations of prison staff. The general message was not to look back at past crimes but forward to a more worthwhile place in society. In sum, the Nicaraguan penal system is one which deserves closer examination, not just because of the option it presents for other developing countries. The use of open and semi-open prisons, as well as the rehabilitation and education programmes, means a lower cost to the community both economically and socially. Prisoners tend not to re-offend, family relationships are maintained, and above all, through education prisoners are provided with the opportunity of a different role in society.

## REFERENCES

Americas Watch (1984) *Human Rights in Nicaragua*, New York.

Amnesty International (1982) *Report of the Amnesty International Missions to the Republic of Nicaragua – August 1979, January 1980, and August 1980*, London.

Catholic Institute for International Relations (1987) *Right to Survive – Human Rights in Nicaragua*, London.

IACHR, Inter-American Commission on Human Rights (1983) *Report on the situation of human rights in the Republic of Nicaragua*, Washington, DC.

*Independent*, 14 March 1989, 'Nicaraguans Told Price of Peace'.

McCabe, B. (1986) Report on recidivism quoted in Central American Historical Institute *Update*, vol. 5, no. 31, 24 July.

# Chapter Seven

# NYKÖPING CLOSED NEIGHBOURHOOD PRISON, SWEDEN

## *NORMAN BISHOP*

## INTRODUCTION

The Howard League's request was for a description of the general characteristics of the Swedish prison system and a more detailed account of a typical Swedish prison taking adult male prisoners. But what is typical? Typical of what? What criteria shall be used to determine typicality? And in what sense can one prison be typical of an entire system?

Let us leave these questions for the moment. In fact, the prison I have chosen to describe is a medium security neighbourhood prison. Explaining why I have chosen such a prison as 'typical' and describing it more closely will make more sense after a general description of imprisonment in Sweden.

## IMPRISONMENT IN SWEDEN

### *Frequency of use*

When compared with the frequency of use of all sanctions, it is apparent from Table 7.1 that imprisonment has been and still is used sparingly.

Of course, the table shows only the relative and proportional use of imprisonment. How many sentenced prisoners are received each year? What is the size of the prison population on average throughout the year?

As Table 7.2 shows, there has been an increase in the number received over the last twenty years but the size of the average prison population has remained fairly stable.

*Table 7.1* Use of various sanctions 1857–1988

| Period | Imprisonment (all forms) % | Fines (all forms) % | Other sanctions % | Number of decisions (annual average) |
|--------|------|------|------|------|
| 1857–60 | 4 | 95 | 1 | 40,996 |
| 1931–35 | 2 | 95 | 3 | 120,362 |
| 1976–80 | 3 | 86 | 11 | 413,983 |
| 1987 | 5 | 84 | 11 | 351,265 |

*Sources:* von Hofer 1983; *Statistics Sweden* 1988

*Table 7.2* Numbers of sentenced prisoners received and average prison population 1970–88

| Year | No. received | Average population | Average no. of days in prison (discharges) |
|------|------|------|------|
| 1975–9 | 11,006 | 3,514 | 104 |
| 1980 | 12,223 | 3,708 | 105 |
| 1981 | 13,296 | 3,912 | 104 |
| 1982 | 13,798 | 4,046 | 105 |
| 1983 | 15,168 | 3,964 | 95 |
| 1984 | 14,647 | 3,534 | 88 |
| 1985 | 15,535 | 3,552 | 96 |
| 1986 | 14,188 | 3,511 | 90 |
| 1987 | 14,980 | 3,643 | 89 |
| 1988 | 16,098* | 3,560* | 81* |

*Note:* The figures for 1975–9 represent an annual average

*Sources: Statistics Sweden* 1988 and *KVS 1989 (preliminary figures for the budget year 1988–9)

### Time in prison and conditional release

The stability of the average population is explained by the fact that most prison sentences are fairly short and that, as the number of receptions has increased in the last nine years, so the average time spent in prison has fallen. Of the 16,000 sentenced prisoners received during 1988, 52 per cent had sentences of up to three months. A further 16 per cent had sentences from three to six months whilst the proportion of those serving from six months up to one year was 17 per cent. For 14 per cent the sentence was one year or longer. Only three persons with life sentences were received during 1988 (KVS forthcoming).

A further factor contributing to the stability of the average prison

131

population are the provisions on conditional release. Conditional release for most prisoners has long been automatically granted after two-thirds of the sentence has been served. However, since July 1983, conditional release on sentences of up to two years is granted after half the sentence has been served providing that a two-month minimum has been completed. Relatively few prisoners are sentenced to more than two years. A special decision is taken on the conditional release of this latter group, but even so, many are released after serving half, or between half and two-thirds of the sentence. Virtually all are released by the time that two-thirds has been served. Even life imprisonment in most cases means only eight to eleven years in prison. (At the time of writing – September 1989 – it seems likely that the two-thirds rule will be re-instituted. It is hoped, however, to reduce the scale of punishment available to the courts for many offences not involving drugs or violence so as to avoid an increase in the average prison population.)

### Offences

What are the offences that have been committed by those that the courts send to prison?

In 1987, 24 per cent of nearly 15,000 receptions had been found guilty of drunken driving, 23 per cent were guilty of some kind of theft, 16 per cent were guilty of crimes of violence, 7 per cent were guilty of serious drug offences, 6 per cent had committed fraud, 3 per cent had been sentenced for offending against military regulations; the remaining 21 per cent had been sentenced for various offences under special legislation, for instance, the Aliens Act. About 11 per cent of prisoners were sentenced in the same judgement for two or more offences carrying similar scales of punishment (KVS 1988).

A sentence to imprisonment for serious drug offences usually means that the offence was trafficking in drugs. Personal drug misuse per se does not lead to imprisonment. Of course, those who traffic in drugs may or may not be drug misusers.

The day-fine system as it is used in Sweden means that for many years now no prisoners have been received for non-payment of fines. Under this system, which is also used in Germany and which, in an adapted form, is now being proposed in England and Wales, the amount of the fine is linked to disposable income and the ability to pay. Thus a particular offence may merit a fine of 30 day units, in the court's view. The actual amount of cash to be paid is determined by calculating the defendant's disposable income after certain essential deductions have been made. The balance, reduced to a daily sum, is then multiplied by the number of days so that the court knows it is within the capacity of the defendant to pay. A defendant on state benefit might finish with a fairly nominal daily sum; a prosperous businessman very much more. The aim is to equalize the impact of the penalty as well as to avoid imprisonment for fine default.

### Types of prison: general organization of the system

If we exclude the remand prisons, there are only two types – neighbourhood prisons and national prisons. Both types can be open or closed. Most closed neighbourhood prisons would, however, be classified internationally as of medium security. Closed national prisons vary; some are of medium security, others are of maximum security.

At the moment, the national prisons come directly under the National Prison and Probation Administration. During the budgetary year 1987–8 there were 1,222 prisoner places in 16 closed national prisons (or closed wings of national prisons) and 472 places in 9 open national prisons (or open wings of national prisons). Sweden's largest national prison, Kumla, has 175 places. Most national prisons have fewer than 100 places. Three national maximum security prisons have special security wings which provide a total of 25 places for particularly dangerous prisoners. National prisons take prisoners serving sentences of more than twelve months as well as prisoners transferred to them for disciplinary or other special reasons.

The neighbourhood prisons (58 of them on 1 July 1988), together with the remand prisons and the probation districts, are grouped in 12 regions under regional directors. Such prisons have only 40 to 60 places. In all, they can accommodate just over 2,200 prisoners.

I have described in detail elsewhere how the present organization of the prison system came into being in 1974 (Bishop 1987). The main reasons underlying the 1974 re-organization were the need to reduce the negative effects of imprisonment and to improve the practical help given to prisoners. To this end, new legislation and

133

new forms of organization were introduced. Both enable prisoners, as far as possible, to serve their sentences near their home communities (the proximity principle) and to have wide opportunities to work or study outside the prison as well as to maintain contact with families and to utilize local social and educational services and cultural and leisure organizations (the normality principle). Generous provision is made for leaves from the prison. In fact, over 43,000 leaves were granted during the budgetary year 1988–9 of which 4 per cent were misused by absconding, late return, intoxicated on return, smuggling attempts, etc.

The prisons which are intended to give special emphasis to the principles outlined here are the neighbourhood prisons. Prisoners sentenced to up to one year's imprisonment are normally placed in them. Prisoners may also be transferred to neighbourhood prisons from national prisons for the terminal part of their time in prison (up to four months) to prepare them for release.

In order to give effect to the proximity and normality principles it was necessary to close a number of older prisons which were ill-adapted to the aims of the re-organized system, and build new neighbourhood prisons. Twenty such prisons have been constructed since 1974.

### Why is a medium security neighbourhood prison 'typical'?

The first reason for choosing to describe a closed neighbourhood prison is quite simply that, numerically speaking, it is representative. This type of prison deals with a larger proportion of received prisoners than any other type of prison. A further reason is that although the closed neighbourhood prisons do not take the most serious or dangerous offenders, they do take prisoners who are criminally experienced and with serious personal and social problems. For instance, the proportion of drug misusers among prisoners received in 1988–9 who were serving a sentence of more than two months and who were known to have been using drugs in the two months prior to their incarceration was 14 per cent in the open national prisons, 27 per cent in the open neighbourhood prisons, 54 per cent in the closed national prisons and 58 per cent in the closed neighbourhood prisons. For all prisons the proportion of drug misusers received was 45 per cent (Krantz and Nilsson 1989).

I chose to describe one of the new neighbourhood prisons because it is typical not only in its prisoner population but also in its architecture, staffing and activities. These new neighbourhood prisons were not constructed solely for male prisoners. In order that women prisoners might have the same opportunities as men prisoners (the small number precludes building special neighbourhood prisons for women), modern neighbourhood prisons have accommodation for both sexes. The women's wings are separated from the men's wings but daytime activities are shared.

I was surprised to be asked to include recidivism figures in the article. In my view it is difficult to see what conclusions can be drawn from them. They can certainly not be used as a measure of the effectiveness of prison rehabilitation measures. Successful resettlement is almost certainly more dependent upon the opportunities afforded to the prisoner on release and the quality of after-care than the assistance given during a brief stay in prison. In any case, no routine recidivism statistics are available by type of prison. A large-scale recidivism study is being undertaken by the Research and Development Group at the National Prison and Probation Administration but no findings are available at present.

## THE NYKÖPING CLOSED NEIGHBOURHOOD PRISON

### Introduction

It is not difficult to come into Nyköping[1] Prison as a visitor if one has some serious purpose in mind. I telephoned the governor, explained why I wanted to visit and was invited to come at once. Of course, I have worked in the prison administration and am known to the governor but earlier this year *Newsweek* had been there and during my visit a San Francisco lawyer telephoned and asked to visit. Permission was given immediately.

### The physical environment

The appearance of the prison, which was built in 1985, is typical of the new neighbourhood prisons. It consists of a two-storey set of buildings in pleasant red brick. It is situated on a main road passing through the industrial area of the town. Despite the double wire fence and barred entrance gate there is little to suggest to the passer-by that this is a prison. It could as well be a factory or office similar to those around it. All buildings are inter-connected and reached by corridors painted and decorated in light colours. Art reproductions hang on the walls and in one long corridor and in the dining room, a local artist has painted attractive murals. There are a number of locked doors at strategic points; these can also be locked from the central control room. The general impression given is more that of a well-equipped hostel than a prison. There is absolutely no prison smell.

There are five rooms for prisoners in each of eight self-contained living units (four units on each floor), in other words, forty prisoners can be accommodated. Each unit has its own set of showers and a small well-equipped kitchen-cum-pantry combined with a breakfast room. There is also a small common room in each unit. Each room has its own toilet separated from the living space in the same way as in most modern hotels. There are no bars on the windows; strengthened laminated glass is used instead. Recreation rooms and a sauna are provided for common use in four of the residential blocks. There is a single large gymnasium. Coin-operated telephones are installed in the inmates' living quarters. In addition to workshops with places for about twenty-five prisoners, rooms are provided for education and training in social and life skills; one of the rooms consists of two well-equipped home kitchens. An office and examination room are provided for the doctor and there is a small sick bay. Two observation rooms can be used to house inmates who, on returning to the prison, are under the influence of alcohol or drugs.

The units, but not the individual prisoners' rooms, are locked up at night. The rooms I saw were clean and quite acceptably tidy. There is no ambition to have quasi-military orderliness in prisoner rooms; they are expected to approximate to normal living circumstances outside prison. The cleaning of the communal areas is a joint responsibility of the prisoners living in that unit.

## Staff

In addition to the governor and a social work assistant, there are 17 basic grade prison officers, 3 principal officers, a chief officer, a workshop chief and 3 workshop instructors, a senior nurse as well as clerical and kitchen staff – 35 persons in all.

## The prisoners

When I visited the prison in September 1989 there were 31 prisoners there. Only one of them was a woman and she was leaving the same day. (I shall later discuss the problems arising when there is a minority of women prisoners in a predominantly male prisoner environment.) About three-quarters of the prisoners come from the town and its environs whilst about one-quarter come from more distant towns in the county or, in some cases, even further afield.

During the budgetary year 1988–9, at least 57 per cent of prisoners received were known to have been using drugs during the two months immediately prior to coming into prison. Three-quarters of these drug misusers were either injecting or taking drugs in some other way daily (Krantz and Nilsson 1989). A minority of prisoners were in prison for the first time; most had either been in prison before or at least been on probation, often three or four times.

## Routines and programmes

On coming to the prison, prisoners spend a week in an introduction unit (one of the five-man units) and are given information about the prison, its rules, its programmes, etc. At the time I visited, a lecture by one of the 'senior' inmates was in progress; he was talking about the week he had just spent at a prison centre, previously a miners' village. This, since being acquired by the National Prison and Probation Administration, is now used for courses, sometimes with the participation of prisoners' families.

Daily routine is as follows. Between 06.30 and 07.30 prisoners are expected to wake up (a clock radio is in each room), prepare and eat breakfast in the living units. Work or study goes on from 7.30 to 12.00, with a fifteen-minute coffee break at 9.30, and one hour for lunch in the scrupulously clean and pleasantly decorated communal cafeteria. Staff and inmates share the same dining-room and food, though staff tend to eat at other times than inmates to avoid queuing. (I ate an excellent lunch there – fried fish fingers, a sauce, good well-peeled potatoes and salad with choice of milk, fruit juice or water to drink, served as attractively as it was prepared.) There are no complaints about food. Work and classes are continued from 13.00 to 16.30 with a fifteen-minute break at 14.45. The evening meal is served in the cafeteria at 17.00. Locking-up time for the living units is at 19.45 but organized leisure activities can continue until 21.30. Room silence is expected after 23.00. The schedule on the weekends allows for getting up and breakfast at the inmate's choice, unlocking of the living unit at 9.00, and similar times for meals as on weekdays.

## Work and study

Seventeen prisoners were in the workshops. Some were doing very simple assembly work – counting out nuts, bolts and washers or measuring out short lengths of flex for electric plugs and putting them in little plastic bags, or filling larger cartons with bags of small components, etc. The work was in no way interesting or challenging. But there was also a variety of machinery (such as lathes and presses) for metal work and a section for industrial painting. Different articles are made depending on the orders that can be secured from outside firms. As part of the current experiments with decentralization, the workshop chief is responsible for securing suitable work and selling the products.

Workshop staff complained bitterly that they were expected to produce good quality work using prisoners who lacked skills and stayed only a relatively short time in the prison (the average is about three months) using machinery which even if it was new when installed, when the prison was opened some four years ago, was old-fashioned. They wanted modern microcomputer-controlled machinery, arguing that this would enable greater prisoner involvement and improve both efficiency and the obtaining of interesting work. Then, they thought, the workshops would be more like those outside prison and therefore a better training. They felt strongly that they did not get adequate support on this matter from regional and central management.

No disciplinary officers were present in the workshops. As one workshop instructor put it, 'We have to see inmates as our work colleagues and secure their collaboration somehow.'

No educational activities were in progress on the day of my visit. However, the municipality provides teachers under the national BASE Scheme (Basic Adult Special Education) and also for training in social and life skills. About five prisoners were involved in these activities, which take place during the afternoon. Another five inmates were engaged for half of the day in a home economics course run by the prison authorities in the well-appointed double kitchen mentioned above. The course lasts five weeks and is apparently much appreciated as a source of home cooking.

Prisoners are paid for both work and study. Average work and study wages are around 350–400 Swedish crowns per week (approximately $55–65).

### Letters, recreation and visits

Prisoners can write as many letters as they wish but must pay the postage themselves. (Postage rates had gone up shortly before my visit. I heard on the day I was at the prison that the local postman was pointing out that prisoners were still using the older, cheaper rates. The local post office was allowing the letters to go through but asked for the matter to be dealt with. One of the staff undertook to bring the matter to the prisoners' notice. I thought that this was an interesting indication of the understanding shown by a local administration.) In general, mail is not examined unless there is reason to suppose that it contains contraband, escape plans, etc. Mail to and from a defence lawyer or Swedish authorities and administrations may not be examined.

In addition to the usual recreational activities (such as table tennis, billiards, television, and organized activities until 21.30) there is provision for extra-mural activities on each weekday evening. Prison officers take small groups of inmates out to football matches, theatre, ice hockey, and so on. The prison's treatment planning board decides which prisoners can take part. Prisoners must be able to show through a urine test that they are 'clean' from drugs before going out on any activity.

As is usual in Swedish prisons, emotional contact and sexual relations between a prisoner and his or her visitor are considered to be private matters for which due provision is made. In consequence, visits take place in private rooms with no staff present. But this policy can lead to drugs being smuggled into the prison. At Nyköping Prison, inmates state on arrival which relatives, or other persons with whom they have close ties, they would like to visit them. Discreet enquiries are made about the potential visitors through the police, the probation office and, possibly, the social welfare services. Criminal and drug-dependent visitors are in general not allowed.

Approved visitors telephone the prison and arrange a suitable time for visiting once a week, with an extra visit possible on the weekend if space allows. Weekday visits are allowed from 17.15 to 19.15 and at two-hour intervals on the weekend beginning at 9.45. Inmates change clothes under supervision before and after a visit and may be searched.

## Drugs

Inmates are routinely urine tested for the presence of cannabis, amphetamines and opiates on arrival and thereafter as necessary to prevent drugs from being smuggled into, or used at, the prison. The analysis of urine samples is an expensive business. Routine analyses make use of an automated process which has a 95 per cent probability of being correct. A higher level of certainty requires a verification by an independent method, which adds to the cost. An analysis for cannabis, the opiates and the amphetamines costs 75 Swedish crowns or about $11. The national bill for urine analyses during the budgetary year 1988–9 was just over 4.3 million Swedish crowns or a little over $650,000. At Nyköping Prison the Governor prefers to make regular use of verification even if this means that, for cost reasons, the number of urine tests must be limited.

During the budgetary year 1988–9, a total of 383 urine tests, including those done on reception, were conducted at Nyköping Prison. Of these, 107 were positive for cannabis, 30 for amphetamines and 7 for opiates. (An inmate can be positive for more than one type of drug.) No conclusions can be drawn from these or similar figures about the extent to which drugs are available or used at the prison. Drugs can and do come into the prison – it would be impossible to prevent this without sealing the prison off completely from society. The Governor believes however that the generous programme of extramural activities and prison leaves, for which freedom from drugs is an essential condition, together with good staff–inmate relations, keeps illicit drugs down to an acceptably low level.

Tests for HIV infection are often conducted at the remand prisons but, during 1988–9, were supplemented by 41 tests at the Nyköping Prison. None was positive but two prisoners were received who had been tested elsewhere and were known to be HIV-positive on arrival.

## Disciplinary infractions and their punishment

Escapes, attempted escapes and drug-related infractions are the commonest reasons for disciplinary reports and punishment. The Prison Treatment Act 1974 provides for only two disciplinary sanctions – a warning and a decision that up to ten days of time in prison shall not count as time served. (There is a maximum aggregation of 45 days for multiple infractions provided that the prisoner is serving more than a four-month sentence.) Over and above the formal disciplinary punishments prisoners may be transferred away, usually to a national prison, as 'unsuitable'.

During the budgetary year 1988–9 about 140 prisoners were received at Nyköping Prison. For the same period, warnings were used on 18 occasions and 'lost time' was used on 50 occasions. There were 13 transfers from the prison for misbehaviour: 7 for escapes or attempted escapes, 4 for repeated drug misuse, one for violence to another inmate and one for repeated alcohol misuse. Not all the disciplinary punishments related to offences in the Nyköping Prison; some prisoners had escaped from another prison and, after apprehension, were re-admitted via Nyköping where they were subject to disciplinary punishment. The Governor, who has himself had experience as a prison officer, is no great believer in formal disciplinary reports. Unless the infractions are serious, he believes that it is better to discuss them, especially those involving conflicts between staff and prisoners. In the four and a half years that the prison has been open there is one recorded instance of violence being used against staff by a prisoner.

## Staff–inmate relations

The governor considers that the level of disciplinary infractions and punishments is acceptably low and attributes this mainly to good staff–inmate relations. As a visitor one gets a general impression of a relaxed but businesslike atmosphere. Prison officers for the most part wear a uniform of blue shirt and blue trousers, sometimes with a tunic. Three or four keys of Yale size open all doors so there is no obvious display of keys. All staff wear a small plastic label showing rank or function and name. Relations between prisoners and staff seemed to be quite informal. In most of the direct conversations that I overheard, first names were used on both sides and I was subsequently told by an inmate that this was very common. Five of the prison's seventeen prison officers are women who perform the same tasks as their male colleagues.

I interviewed one of these women prison officers who, at the time of my visit, was in charge of the ground floor living units. She gave an immediate impression of friendly capability. Her earlier work experience had been in the health service but, on the advice of a friend, she had decided to try the prison service. She told me that a woman prison officer among mostly male inmates is subjected to a good deal of testing-out. Prisoners want to see if they can 'get away' with behaviour which would not be tolerated by a man. Some of the testing-out takes the form of trying to find out about the private life of a woman prison officer. It was absolutely necessary to find ways of setting limits, she considered. Once this had been achieved she thought that she had no more difficulty in handling inmates or dealing with difficult situations than male officers. Sensitivity enters into this, however, as the following example shows.

Like her male colleagues she is required from time to time to supervise the taking of urine samples. To avoid faked samples the inmate must be naked when urinating and under close observation. Women prison officers are not excused from taking their turn at this duty, one which even many male prison officers find unpleasant. 'I know,' she said, 'that for many foreign prisoners it is shameful to be observed by a woman in this situation. And it would be hard for them to tell me so. I may have to do it anyway, but there are times when I try to arrange for a male colleague to do it instead to spare a foreign prisoner's feelings.'

She is convinced that women prison officers can make a unique contribution. One prisoner took no interest in his personal hygiene and was resistant to the attempts of male prison officers and other inmates to get him to wash and shower more often. But when my interviewee told him that he must do so he complied willingly. She also said, 'Prisoners come very often to us women to talk about worries and difficulties with wives, girl-friends, children and other very personal problems. It seems that they do not find it so easy to talk with men about such matters.' But some male prison officers have reservations about the usefulness of women prison officers, 'so, if you are a woman, you have to prove that you can do the job one hundred and twenty per cent!' This means that she and her female colleagues talk a good deal with each other about the job and its difficulties.

This woman prison officer is active in a working group which is drawing up plans to present to the Governor about creating completely drug-free living units. Prisoners would apply to enter these units and agree to intensive urine testing. Being drug free would entitle them to a range of extra privileges and benefits.

In describing this project she said, 'It would be better for the prisoners and better for us on the staff. After all, the prison is our working environment as well as the place where prisoners work and live. I think we all have a right to be free from this pest.' (The Governor approves of this planning, which he also sees as an important way of increasing staff involvement in the work of the prison.)

I asked if she liked the work. Did it offer job satisfaction? She said that she had been two years at the prison and despite all the difficulties found the work deeply satisfying. In fact, this was obvious from her whole attitude and manner; my question was really superfluous.

### A prisoner's views

I also interviewed a prisoner (the one who had been lecturing to new inmates in the introduction wing). He was 55 years old and had at one time been sentenced to the now-abolished indeterminate sentence of internment, which was intended for seriously recidivist offenders. He had seen the inside of a good many prisons since his career began in the 1950s. He thought the Nyköping Prison offered decent living conditions and that prisoners were treated by the staff as human beings. There were good opportunities for work, education and leisure. He had seen over the years how drugs had come to influence the lives of prisoners whilst they were in prison. He told me what has been well documented in research (Åkerström 1985, 1986) – that even in the Nyköping Prison it was often necessary for new prisoners to be able to prove to others on arrival that they had not been informers to the police, prosecutor or the court about others involved in drug trafficking. There was, in his view, not much wrong with the prison or its staff; it was the involvement of inmates with drugs that was the problem. Threats and debts because of drugs were what he deplored most. They might not be common but even limited blackmailing pressures were bad for the inmate community. The five-man living units could be bad from this point of view 'though after the introduction week everyone usually gets some choice of living unit and can find others he gets along with'.

### The inmate council

Prisoners have a right in law to discuss together matters of common interest and present their views to the Governor. On alternate Thursdays the prisoners hold a community meeting unattended by staff. An elected inmate council meets the Governor on the other alternate Thursdays if there are proposals to put forward or grievances to be discussed on behalf of the prisoner collective.

### Criticisms

There is a danger that my picture of this prison makes it look too good. Perhaps so – but, in my view, there is little doubt that a prison of this kind does make a serious and by no means unsuccessful attempt to remove some of the negative effects of imprisonment. This is not to say that there is no room for criticism. And a number of features of the prison which look good at first sight reveal themselves on closer examination to have disadvantages or to present problems.

The criticisms of the workshop instructors have been mentioned above. In short, they consider that with modern computer-regulated machinery and improved support from central or regional management they could secure better orders and achieve better selling. In their view this would heighten prisoner interest in work and enhance the training effect of work. Present legislation makes it obligatory for prisoners to work or study if fit. The workshop staff would like to see this obligation abolished. Instead they would like to see a minimum wage paid to all prisoners regardless of whether they worked and studied. But for those who did work and study there would be substantially increased wages.

The interview with the prisoner suggested that it is by no means certain that the five-man living units are wholly beneficial in character. The Governor concurred with this view. The staff on duty must keep an eye on all the activities in the prison and cannot give so much time to the living units. They visit the units but do not work in close and continuous contact with the prisoners in them. Then, too, the living units are locked up at 19.45 and the prisoners are left in contact with each other. There are positive aspects to this – prisoners need not experience 'cell terror' by being locked in. If they cannot sleep they can get up and make a sandwich or a drink in the pantry or talk to a mate. On the other hand, though, it is easy for the group to talk crime, plan escapes or drug deals and put pressure on weaker members of the group.

One consequence of the 1974 re-organization was a reduction of the earlier procedures and possibilities for prisoner differentiation. The advantages of neighbourhood prisons were thought to out-weigh the possible disadvantages of grouping different kinds of prisoner together. In the light of fifteen years' experience, which includes an increasing awareness of the part played by drugs and drug trafficking in the life of the prison community, there is reason to ask if a greater measure of differentiation now needs to be provided. This would mean making it possible to differentiate so that, for example, women prisoners were not a small minority in a neighbourhood prison where young and old, experienced and in-experienced offenders, drug misusers and non-drug misusers tend to be mixed together. There are current plans to reduce the number of regions and to incorporate the national prisons in the new regions. These plans are part of a scheme for reducing the decision-making powers of the central administration in favour of a far-reaching decentralization of the prison system. But another aim is to improve possibilities for differentiation of prisoners.

At Nyköping Prison the Governor thinks that this is especially necessary for women prisoners. It is undoubtedly positive that the much smaller number of women prisoners can have access to fami-lies and local social services, etc., in the same way as men. Before 1974 all women prisoners served their sentences in the only women's prison that existed in Sweden and many were therefore great distances from their homes. On the other hand there may be only one or two women prisoners and thirty or more men prisoners in a neighbourhood prison. The women prisoners under these circumstances can be unhealthily dominated by some of the men and relationships which are damaging to both partners grow up.

At Nyköping Prison the staff have seen an 18-year-old girl become attracted to an older drug misuser and marry him despite all efforts to ensure waiting until after release from prison to test the relation-ship. The history of the pair after their release has been one of wife-beating, separation and the taking into care of the couple's child. They have seen a number of similar unhappy examples. A neighbourhood prison for women prisoners only has recently been started in the Stockholm region and is attempting to deal with the special problems of women prisoners. The experiment is being evaluated.

Another point is of general nature, but was also mentioned at the Nyköping Prison. The 1974 re-organization emphasized the import-ance of the responsibility of the probation services in planning for the release of prisoners. The probation services were also intended to initiate co-ordinated action by other relevant social services as part of this preparation. So the probation services had to be in close contact with prisoners in the neighbourhood prisons and with a network of social services. In practice, it has proved difficult to achieve what was originally hoped. Effective co-operation has been hampered by the fact that each organization is governed by its own rules and regulations (and these are not always understood outside that organization), conflicts can occur and, within the probation services, there have been many staff changes and resignations. If there is no fully efficient collaboration with and between local probation and social services the work of a neighbourhood prison is seriously jeopardized. The government's attention has been drawn to this problem by the National Prison and Probation Adminis-tration in its budgetary request for 1990–1. Whatever the outcome of that initiative the Governor of Nyköping Prison is urging that joint treatment planning meetings should be held between repre-sentatives of the probation service, the labour exchange, the social services, etc. He considers joint treatment planning to be especially necessary for prisoners with particularly difficult social circum-stances or personal handicaps.

As a final note on criticisms I should like to add the following. It seemed to me that there was a good deal of healthy self-criticism among the staff I met at the Nyköping Prison. The critical views that they expressed were often well reasoned and followed by ideas on improvements. Much of the criticism brought forward and des-cribed briefly above has also often been documented in two lengthy research reports on the functioning of neighbourhood prisons published by the National Prison and Probation Administration itself (Krantz, Pettersson and Bishop 1981, Krantz and Pettersson 1984). Why, asked the staff I spoke with, does no one listen to us? Why do we have to adjust to a number of changes conceived at the central administration which seem to us to take no account of the reality we see and deal with? And when everyone can see that there is an obvious weakness in something we are doing, why does it take so long to effect change? Why, for example, have twenty new prisons been built, every one with its five-man living units when everyone can see that there are problems around the idea? Why, they asked, have we not experimented to keep what is good in the idea and get over some of the difficulties?

These are not only good questions which demand answers. They are also an indication of a potential among the staff for growth and change in an effort to reduce still further the damaging effects of imprisonment. As such they deserve to be taken seriously. Not to do so is to create cynicism and apathy. In the world generally there are disturbing pressures which make for ever larger prison populations, more and more prisons and harsher prison conditions.There have been real attempts in Sweden, I believe, to resist these pressures. The prison I have described is a part of that attempt. The future, as always, is an open question. But choice plays a part in the future that becomes the present. Will we go on or go back? The only certain thing is that we cannot stand still.

## NOTE

1 Nyköping is pronounced as 'noo-sherp-ing', with even accentuation of the three syllables.

## REFERENCES

Åkerström, M. (1985) *Violence and threats among prison inmates*. Report no. 1985: 2 (Swedish only), Research and Development Group, KVS, S-601 80 Norrköping.
—— (1986) 'Outcasts in prison: the case of informers and sex offenders', in *Deviant Behaviour* 7: 1–12, Hemisphere Publishing Corporation.
Bishop, N. (1987) 'A present-day prison system: structural and functional requirements', in symposium report, *The Centenary of Deprivation of Liberty in The Netherlands*, The Hague: Ministry of Justice. Also published in *Council of Europe Prison Information Bulletin* 7, July 1986.

NORMAN BISHOP

Hofer, H. von (1983) *Brott och straff 1 Sverige 1750–1982 (Crime and punishment in Sweden 1750–1982)*, *Statistics Sweden* (a Swedish government publication) 115 81 Stockholm.

Krantz, L. and Nilsson, M. (1989) *Drug misusing prisoners during the financial year 1988–9*, forthcoming report (Swedish and English), Norrköping: Research and Development Group, KVS, S-601 80.

Krantz, L. and Pettersson, T. (1984) *New neighbourhood prisons: follow-up interviews four years later*, Report no. 1984:1 (Swedish only), Norrköping: Research and Development Group, KVS, S-601 80.

Krantz, L., Pettersson, P. and Bishop, N. (1981) *New neighbourhood prisons: the initial phase at Orretorp, Tygelsjö, Helsingborg and Luleå prisons*, Report no. 35, (Swedish only), Norrköping: Research and Development Group, KVS, S-601 80.

KVS (1988) *Annual Report of the National Prison and Probation Administration* (abbreviated to KVS in Swedish) for the budgetary year 1987–8 (English summary), S-601 80 Norrköping.

KVS (forthcoming) *Annual Report for the budgetary year 1988–9 of the National Prison and Probation Administration* (abbreviated to KVS in Swedish) (English summary), S-601 80 Norrköping.

*Statistics Sweden* (1988) *Yearbook of Judicial Statistics* (a Swedish government publication), Stockholm.

# Chapter Eight

# GEURRERO CENTRE FOR REHABILITATION, MEXICO

## *BRIAN SMITH*

Mexico is a country with over three thousand years of continuous civilization, but knowledge of its history, culture and people has tended to be either minimal or – worse – affected by the kind of stereotypes we acquire from film or television. People and even nations are often pigeon-holed according to people's preconceived ideas, which are of course seldom accurate. This is certainly the fate of the Mexican people. I have visited Mexico on a number of occasions and seen both major cities and rural areas. In both, a warm, dignified and considerate people provide a marked contrast to the simple peasants or scruffy bandits who are all too often seen on screen.

As a magistrate on the Nottingham bench, I had visited a number of English prisons and young offenders' institutions during the weeks immediately before my visit to Mexico. I would not claim specialist knowledge of penal systems in Britain or overseas but offer my observations as those of an interested and reasonably informed member of the general public.

I last visited Mexico for almost a month during May and June 1989. I chose to try to see the system and situation in a more rural area of Mexico. The country is divided into thirty-two states which are in many respects self-governing, with laws differing from state to state, although all are subject to the national federal law.

The area I visited, Geurrero State, is in the south-west coastal area of Mexico and includes that idyll of jet-setters – Acapulco. It was from there that I began my efforts to enquire into the operation of the judicial system in the area. My interest was entirely personal and motivated by my recent visits to, and my impressions of, the English prisons and young offenders' institutions.

It took almost three days to make the appointments necessary to meet three local judges. Until recently very few Europeans and hardly anyone from England had visited this area and they did not appear to have had any previous requests from foreign visitors for information, visits to courts or access to their prisons. I had taken a letter of introduction from my own bench and from the Magistrates Association. Without at least some form of official introduction it would have been almost impossible to get the co-operation and approval necessary to visit any government penal centre or institution.

The three judges I met included the first woman judge to be appointed in Geurrero State. I was most impressed by their apparent concern for the individual and his or her rights. Ample opportunity appeared to exist for local people to obtain free advice on basic legal problems. A constant flow of people was being seen by various clerks and secretaries, while at regular intervals one or other of the judges would be called away to advise on a particular problem or situation. Because of the way in which my visit to the judges and the prison was arranged, I am quite confident that no 'set-piece' situations or activities had been organized just for my benefit or to create a more favourable impression of the judicial system or the detention centre.

The basis for the Mexican legal system is the Napoleonic Code which means a supposition of guilt until proved otherwise. My first reaction to this basic precept was that it must be a difficult and sometimes hopeless task for the average 'campesino' (worker) to cope with. Despite the fact that the Mexican government spends almost 25 per cent of its budget on education, a high proportion of the population is still relatively poor, semi-literate and ill-equipped to grasp even the fundamentals of the legal system, let alone to take it on in what would appear to be a very one-sided battle against the establishment and its administration. That they have managed to cope with it at all is perhaps some credit to at least a reasonable level of fairness within the system. The prisons do not appear to be full to overflowing as in so many European countries. There are not constant outcries against the police, courts and prisons, so perhaps the Code works in a sufficiently balanced way, so as to blend at least reasonably well with the democracy so fervently fought for in Mexico's history.

The judicial system is at the primary level operated by locally appointed judges who seemed to have very similar power and jurisdiction to English magistrates. The next level are in fact magistrates, who appear to have a similar area of responsibility to our Crown Court judges. Finally there are federal judges, who have a general and overriding authority over the other levels of jurisdiction. They also handle those cases concerned with major crime or of national concern and interest.

As far as I could discern none of the courts operates on any form of jury system. All cases are handled by one of the three levels of jurisdiction, someone usually sitting alone. An arrested person must be brought before a judge within forty-eight hours, who will then decide if there is a case to answer. If so the alleged offender may be held in custody to await trial. In Geurrero State this waiting period was apparently not too long but it appeared that in other areas delays and crowded court lists inevitably meant some people spending a considerable time in custody.

Defendants who do not have their own lawyer may select one, from a list, who will then represent them entirely free of charge. However, these state lawyers tend in many cases to be the newest and very often amongst the least experienced in the profession. The prosecution is handled by the state.

On the morning of my visit the courts were only dealing with a limited number of very minor matters, mostly drink related. These resulted in fairly short sentences to the local prison, often of only 3 to 7 days, or up to 3 months for the more habitual drink offender. The Mexicans seem to be following a general trend in renaming their penal institutions, and many prisons are now referred to as 'Centres for Rehabilitation'.

One of the judges agreed to accompany me on a visit to one of these centres. The Geurrero Centre for Rehabilitation is located in a comparatively deserted, rugged area of the mountainous region some thirty to fifty kilometres from Acapulco.

The first impression was, to say the least, somewhat awe inspiring – smooth, dark grey, concrete walls stretching up about ten metres with raised gun-towers approximately every 100 metres. These were manned by guards whose only access to the towers was by way of a single rope which they had to climb in a gymnastic fashion; they then pulled up the rope and remained in the towers for the rest of the shift. They could therefore spend a considerable period of time in the towers, in full uniform, in temperatures of anything up to 100 degrees Fahrenheit, or more. Virtually all the guards carried at least a side-arm and, usually, a semi-automatic rifle. I questioned the need

151

for such a display of guns and they seemed to find it difficult to justify them. It certainly did not appear to be because they had any great fear of violence or mass escapes. The guards were apparently not given any regular weapons training and I felt that they really carried the weapons more as part of their uniform and tradition than because of absolute necessity. The group I talked to could only recall one prisoner escaping in recent years; he had been shot during his escape and even then was not recaptured.

Admission into the complex followed a similar pattern to that I had seen in the English prisons: searches, registration, allocation, different coloured uniforms for the various categories of prisoner, etc. I met the governor – although he is now more generally called the 'Principal', apparently in keeping with the educational and rehabilitative emphasis which this particular centre tried to use with its inmates. As we walked around the complex, the Principal dressed informally in shirt sleeves, no guns or armed guards with us at all, the whole atmosphere appeared to be very relaxed. Many of the prisoners smiled and exchanged a few words either directly with the governor or with people in our party. Despite this I still had a strong impression that the Principal was clearly in control of the centre and that he would be unlikely to tolerate breaches of the rules.

A noticeable feature of the Geurrero Centre was the relative freedom the inmates had to move within quite large areas of the complex. But access outside their own particular areas was only achieved by those issued with special access cards that had to be signed by one of the guards. A very limited number of guards was apparent around the centre. Considering the extensive area the complex covered and the large and varied number of the inmates, considerably more guards or prison officers might have been expected, with a much more rigid control over the movements and integration of the prisoners.

The Principal offered me complete freedom to visit and photograph any part of the complex. It occupies an area of approximately 20 hectares and includes an administration block for the courts and associated administrative staff. Men, women and juveniles are all housed in the same complex, although in segregated areas. The centre can accommodate up to 2,000 inmates at any one time.

The centre is almost entirely self-sufficient, growing a wide variety of crops, raising animals – it included a very sophisticated pig breeding and rearing programme – and literally hundreds of rabbits and

152

chickens. A number of large and efficiently run workshops made a wide range of products for use in the centre and for sale in nearby towns. I was most impressed with the quality, variety and complexity of some of the items prisoners were making and the apparent pride they had in the quality of workmanship. The work did not appear to be just one of those relatively soul destroying, 'anything to keep them occupied' jobs that many prison inmates are forced to undertake. The prisoners were actually making complete items of furniture, doors, window frames, pottery and jewellery. They also made most of the furniture and fittings used in the prison buildings. I understand that they were working to commissioned orders for a very wide range of goods and products, which were then sold in government-run shops in local towns. The proceeds were used to maintain, run and develop the prison. All the buildings I saw in the complex were well maintained, clean, light and well ventilated.

The female inmates were mainly employed in a domestic capacity as cleaners, cooks, etc., or in the laundry. Women made up only a minor proportion of the prison population in Geurrero and I was assured that this situation was reflected throughout Mexico.

The prisoners are allowed out of their cells from around 5.30 in the morning until 6.30 in the evening, during which time a majority of them would be involved in some type of work; this is because for every two days they work they can earn one day's remission of sentence. I was told that they receive three meals a day and a very small amount of payment, although this did not appear to be directly related to the amount of work they did.

I did not have an opportunity to see any meals being served whilst I was there so I cannot be sure of either the quality or quantity. On my way out, however, I saw dozens of plastic bags full of fruit and other food, which had been left by family and friends for the prisoners. This extra food seems to have been provided more as a gesture by the family, than as basic sustenance.

Ample time is allowed for sport and recreation and various football pitches, basketball courts and other facilities were dotted around the complex. There was even a well equipped playground which could have been dropped into any English park almost unnoticed but which looked rather incongruous in the centre of a Mexican prison complex.

Basic education now seems to play an increasingly important part in the rehabilitation of offenders. The Geurrero Centre apparently made every effort to ensure that all the inmates received at least some form of educational tuition during the period of their sentence. Those inmates classed as illiterate were obliged to take a compulsory form of basic education, with the aim that they would at least be able to read and write by the time they were released. Those offenders taking part in this more intense form of education were also expected to work, not towards a reduction in their sentence, but in order to support the education they were receiving. This was apparently reasonably well received by the offenders involved, as even this basic standard of education would be sufficient to improve considerably their potential for employment and thus for higher earnings after their release. I was told that the incidence of re-offending was very low but I was not given any actual figures in support of this.

Cell accommodation is divided into single or two-storey blocks, each comprising 60 to 80 cells of approximately 2m in width and 3 to 4m long, with a barred, 'gate-type' door at each end. This allows at least a reasonable throughput of air; the mid-day temperatures are usually around 80 to 100°F, sometimes more. Each cell housed two or, in some cases, three people. There was little or no evidence of 'home comforts' in the cells, the walls of which were plain concrete, with cot-type beds and what really amounted to a hole in the wall to house each occupant's personal effects. The only forms of decoration were photographs of family, children and, in a majority of cells, some form of religious symbol, usually a picture or statue of 'Our Lady of Guadalupe'.

The cells did not have any form of integral sanitation and each block had a central toilet and shower unit. At the time of my visit virtually all the cells were open and those prisoners in them were free to move around, certainly in the area of their own cells and blocks.

Virtually all the inmates I saw and spoke to were friendly, smiling and quite pleased to show me the work they were doing. I certainly felt much more at ease moving around this institution by myself than I did when visiting some English prisons and institutions. There was certainly not the constant locking, unlocking and clanging of doors nor was there the feeling of oppression that is so often felt when moving around most prisons.

The oppressive regime I had anticipated was not apparent and the whole complex seemed clean, active and designed as far as possible to provide reasonable conditions and amenities for its inmates. There were, however, no signs of television, a cinema or the usual indoor recreations. Visitors are allowed on Thursdays and Sundays for just thirty minutes. I was assured, though, that this time is seldom adhered to, with most visitors remaining for most of the afternoon.

After this visit to the Geurrero Centre, I discussed the prison and its regime with people both inside and outside the criminal justice process. Geurrero cannot be described as 'typical' in that it does not include the most serious offenders, including those convicted of serious violence or large-scale drug offences. But it does illustrate the trend towards the rehabilitation of offenders which the Mexican authorities seem to be making, and the increasing efforts which are being put in towards improving accommodation and educational facilities.

# Chapter Nine

# GELDERN PRISON, FEDERAL REPUBLIC OF GERMANY[1]

## CHRISTIAN KUHN

What is the situation of many of the so-called 'criminals'? Behind peep-holes, between bed and toilet, with the knowledge that they are left alone with their problems, and abandoned. Their labour they see as hard labour, their sentence seems too high and un-justified. The worst for them is to feel that they are powerless in the hands of an omnipotent system. Immediately the prisoner arrives he has to strip in front of the guards, to bow down for inspection, to clean himself and then to be dressed in the prison clothes. Inmates say that they have to leave their personality at this moment in the deposit room. Things that are important, even essential, to them are taken from them. Whatever they do, the whole day is under control and regulation. Each favour has to be requested in writing. Sentence is not only detention. The inmate is losing all right of self-determination or self-government so that he feels that finally his own life is not anymore owned by himself. Decisions are taken about him. He is accommodated in a very small room, without any possibility of privacy, surrounded by fences and walls. The inmate feels like a second- or third-class-man . . .

This (a close translation) is part of an article in the inmate newspaper *Die Posaune* (*The Trombone*), brought out in the prison of Geldern in Nordrhein-Westfalen, Federal Republic of Germany. It is a reflection on the prison situation. The execution of a punishment must by its nature be an evil. Yet can it, despite its destructive elements, help to solve the problems of those concerned? Does it try, as far as possible, to keep the dignity of each one afflicted by it? These are questions which have to be answered not only by the penal system as a whole, but also by each prison within it.

I shall be trying to describe life in the German prison of Geldern, as far as it is possible to do so after having spent one week there. Of course this description is incomplete and subjective, but it will be an attempt to focus on some central points.

Geldern Prison was built in the 1970s and became operational in 1979. It has space for 551 adult male inmates. This is a so called *geschlossener Vollzug*, for serious offenders (a closed penitentiary, as distinct from the *offener Vollzug* – open penitentiary). The average age of the inmates is about 27 years and there are about 30 prisoners serving life sentences. In this prison there are no terrorists and few foreigners.

The ground plan of the prison is like a comb: four parallel wings with two or three floors each, containing the cells. The wings are connected by a building containing administration and workrooms. Twelve 'departments' or prison wings each have 52 single rooms and one four-bedded room for the inmates. On 10 July 1989 there were 490 inmates.

The responsibility of implementing prison sentences lies with the individual states within the Federal Republic of Germany. The state of Nordrhein-Westfalen started a process of penal reform in the late 1970s with the intention 'to re-incorporate the offender into society' and 'to enable the prisoner to live without becoming liable to further prosecution'. Therefore, in the words of the Minister of State, Herr Krumsiek, it requires social training to enable prisoners to become 'more self-responsible, self-confident and active'.

The number of prisoners in Nordrhein-Westfalen has reduced from about 18,000 in 1984 to about 14,000 in 1988. The ministry has consequently reduced the number of available cells for inmates by changing the cells in the prison of Werl into living units with kitchens so that the prison lost some of its 800 capacity. There has also been an emphasis on the development of open prisons; Nordrhein-Westfalen now has 3,700 places in such institutions, which is almost half the total for the Federal Republic of Germany. The state also uses '*Urlaub*', or home leave periods, in order to try to counteract the problems of isolation from the home environment which inevitably arise in prison.

Prisoners come to Geldern after they have spent some time in one of the two special prisons for allocation. After his arrival in Geldern a plan for the remainder of his sentence is worked out, based on discussions of his personal situation, the wishes of the prisoner and the possibilities available. The prisoner has the right to discuss his wishes personally with the warden, or Governor. There are good educational opportunities, at an advanced level, but these are not compulsory. There are other work options, too.

### Vocational training and work

Education and vocational training are what Geldern Prison is all about, and it provides this facility for the whole state. For this, inmates of other prisons transfer to Geldern, even those who would not normally be obliged to be in a closed prison. The training centre was planned and established at the very beginning of the life of the prison. Now, long-term inmates have the chance of a solid training and more and more are given the opportunity at the beginning of a long sentence.

Three parties are involved in the programme: the Ministry of Justice, the Labour Exchange (promotion, provision of machinery) and the group 'Reso' (Resozialisation) of the unions. The manager of the training centre remarked that on several occasions claims have been made by the public that inmates are educated on the most modern and expensive machinery while 'outside' a lot of young people are unable to find a job.

About half of the prison capacity, that is, 220 places, are available in the education centre. During July 1989, 167 inmates were so involved, while another 34 took part in a special course in order to complete their primary school education (an eight-year period) and be prepared for their trade or profession. Twelve different 'craftsmen' jobs are taught in the education centre, in courses lasting about 18 months each (40 hours a week, two-thirds practice and one-third theory). Finally the graduate gets a skilled worker certificate, which does not show that he has had his training in a prison. Foreigners who are to be deported after sentence do not get this training because of the criteria for selection imposed by the labour exchange. Since the centre began more than 1,000 prisoners have passed through, and 78 per cent of them completed their training course.

The inmates participating in the training programme are housed separately from the other prisoners, in two of the four wings. Their regime is different from that of the other prisoners; the rules concerning leisure time are, for instance, more liberal, with cell doors open until 21.00, so that everybody is free to move around. In the other wings the inmates are much more restricted. The atmosphere also seems different in the training centre. There are no problems in this group over personal cleanliness, but the problem can arise with the other prisoners. When electing deputies (the inmates elect 'speakers' who have some sort of shared responsibility for the prison regime) the voting rate of the inmates involved in the training programme was about 70 per cent while for the other inmates, it was only about 40 per cent. This significant difference illustrates the variation between the two wings. If necessary, the training programme can take precedence over penal measures (for example, if solitary confinement is imposed it can be served during the weekends so as not to disturb the training course).

In general all inmates work in the prison and there is enough work for all inmates. On 7 July 1989 about sixty inmates were not at work through illness, refusal, or lack of ability.

There is a large metal-processing workshop which prepares motors for an outside company and pays very good salaries (up to DM 300 per month) but also requires hard work. There is a printing workshop, a chip-processing workshop and several domestic services including the kitchen and laundry.

A small number of prisoners are simply not able to cope with the work environment and for them a special training course is run, with the aim of giving basic work skills and disciplines and enabling them to become accustomed to the working week. When I visited, some six prisoners were participating in this course.

The working day lasts eight hours and the payment to the inmate is about DM 9 ($5) per day. Prisoners pay 1.5 per cent of their salary for unemployment insurance, but they do not have any social security insurance – though they would like to have it. This point is made regularly by the prisoners' representatives.

Half the salary can be used to buy food from the prison shop and the other half is put aside for the time of release. At their request, interest may be paid to the prisoners on this part of their money. Three weeks per year the inmate is free not to work. The inmate newspaper claims that during this 'holiday' period the breakfast is not as good as that provided when prisoners are at work.

CHRISTIAN KUHN

*The daily routine*

Working days:

05.45  Wake up (Reveille)
06.00  Cells are unlocked
06.30  Breakfast
06.50  Prisoners go to work
07.00  Work starts
10.00  Refreshment
10.15  Work continues
11.45  Return to cells
12.00  Lunch
12.45  Work resumes
16.00  End of work
16.30  Exercise
17.30  Showers, change of laundry
18.00  Dinner
18.30  Start of leisure, or free time
21.00  End of leisure time
22.00  Day ends

Electricity remains on in the ceils after 22.00 for the radio, lamp and water heater.

On weekends and holidays reveille is one hour later and the day may be spent in leisure activities or as free time.

*Leisure time*

One hour a day is allowed for exercise. There are four courtyards, partly grassed. Besides this there is a soccer ground, some smaller sporting facilities, a large gymnasium and other training facilities. About ten prisoners, at the time of my visit, were excluded from recreational activities for reasons of security.

About 80 per cent of the inmates are active in sport. Soccer, volley-ball, table tennis and basketball are played. Every year twelve prisoners are trained to become soccer referees, and they then take charge of matches within the prison. This referee training is conducted at a professional level, so the inmate is able to continue it after release; it provides practical help in social integration and may also help with attitudes to authority, the acceptance of discipline, and in accepting criticism. Matches are regularly organized with

160

teams from other prisons, with outside groups and with the guards. Two staff members are responsible, full time, for sporting activities. Two table tennis teams take part in the county championship and they play about forty matches a year in the gymnasium at the prison.

The prison has a library with about 8,000 books; it also boasts a rock band and a range of courses covering handicrafts, interaction-experience, creative painting, and literature. An exhibition of paintings by the prisoners raised money which has been given to a charity founded by the parents of children suffering from cancer.

During the prisoners' free time a range of voluntary activities is available covering alcohol problems (with Alcoholics Anonymous) and special counselling for drug-addicted prisoners or those diagnosed as HIV-positive.

About ninety of the prisoners are married and since April 1988, a marriage counsellor has worked in the prison. In December 1988 about fifteen couples were able to spend an afternoon together with their children celebrating a so-called *Familiennachmittag*, or family get-together.

### Life in the prison

My overall impression was of a very organized institution. The food is adequate in quantity and the quality satisfying, with special diets for Muslims, invalids and vegetarians. Prisoners have about 780 gm of fresh fruits each week.

Visitors from outside are allowed twice each month for an hour's visit. More extended visits are possible and often granted. The visiting rooms are relatively small, however, and the connection to public transport rather poor, involving a bus journey and a walk. Many complaints concern the fact that there is no shelter for visitors waiting outside the prison before they are allowed in for visits. Only an old shelter protects against the rain.

Since the autumn of 1989 three special 'long-term visiting rooms' have been available. There prisoners are able to meet without supervision, providing the visitors are family members (parents, children) or their wives (providing they have been married at least six months). The rooms were nearly finished when I visited. They are in effect small flats, with sitting and cooking facilities, toilet and shower. They have a special entrance, separated from the entrance used by other visitors. Since such facilities are for conjugal visits, they need to be sympathetically and sensitively arranged and from what I saw, that will be achieved very well.

The plan to develop such facilities came after a delegation of parliamentarians of Nordrhein-Westfalen had paid a visit to the prison of Barcelona. They were impressed with what they saw and instructed their own Minister of State to create similar facilities in some of the prisons for which they are responsible.

Three times a year each prisoner is allowed to receive a parcel with food and tobacco from outside: at Christmas and Easter (weighing 3 kg each) and once at a time of his choice (of 5 kg). HIV-positive prisoners can receive a monthly food parcel. These prisoners are integrated into the ordinary life of the prison, not separated from the other prisoners, but only work where there is a minimum risk of injury. If any develop AIDS, they are transferred to hospital.

Hard drugs are not of particular importance in the prison, but cannabis, or hashish, plays a significant role. About 30 per cent of the inmates are reported to have used it. Prison staff are constantly trying to control drug abuse, with urine sampling, regular cell changes (to minimize concealment) and surprise searches. That they have had some success is demonstrated by the price of a gramme of cannabis, which has risen to DM 40 ($20) from between DM 20 and DM 30. The latter price is the one which obtains in most other prisons, according to information provided by an inmate, and is not very different from the ordinary street price. The relatively high price in Geldern indicates that cannabis is not easily and everywhere available. Alcohol is strictly prohibited throughout the prison.

Disciplinary measures, strictly regulated by law, range from restrictions on leisure time, shopping and visits, to solitary confinement for a maximum of four weeks. During solitary confinement, the exercise period for the prisoner can be cancelled and this often happens. Solitary confinement is imposed about 40 times a year, restrictions on shopping in about 70 cases, restrictions on leisure in about 250 cases. In an emergency the inmate can be physically secured to a bed (*Fesselbrett*), but this is, for all practical purposes, not in use. If used, the Governor has to report the fact after three days to a higher authority.

Self-inflicted injury is rare and does not seem to be used to put pressure on staff to achieve a prisoner's particular demands. The statistics for 1988 record two cases of self-injury and five of refusal of food. Since the opening of the prison in 1979 there has been one case of suicide.

According to law the prisoner can have up to 21 days a year on 'Urlaub' (home leave). He can leave the prison providing that the balance of his sentence is less than 18 months. In Geldern up to a third of the inmates are entitled to this benefit. In 1988 there were 2,200 requests for 'Urlaub'; 1,250 were granted. The rate of those failing to return punctually was 2 per cent.

A full-time doctor takes care of the medical service. In discussion with inmates the question was raised as to whether the diagnoses were always careful enough, but prisoners who are seriously ill are in any case transferred to a hospital run by the justice department (at Froendenberg) or to a public hospital. Specialist doctors visit the prison regularly or prisoners may be escorted to facilities in the community. The process for making a complaint is regulated by law and prisoners are carefully informed about their rights.

There is an establishment of seven posts for social workers, but in fact only six are filled at present. Similarly, only two of the three positions for psychologists are filled. The reason is that vacancies must remain unfilled for six months for economic reasons. One of the social workers claimed that he and his colleagues have to use much of their time for administrative work: progress reports or comments, in cases where conditional release or parole is being considered. He himself had to prepare no fewer than 432 reports in 1988. This takes so much time that there may not be time enough for the social work needs of prisoners. He questioned whether, under these conditions, the work can be handled in a satisfactory way.

There seemed to be no particularly strong 'subculture' and relatively few cases of violence between prisoners. That was confirmed by an inmate who had been imprisoned for twelve years and had been in two other prisons before coming to Geldern. In describing Geldern Prison in a generally positive way he claimed that the possibilities for illegal or uncontrolled activities were too few. The situation is different in each wing and, according to a senior prison officer, there are inmates who live in fear. But there seemed to be no large, organized, subcultural structure of power or tyranny.

The reason may be not only the strict control the prison regime has but also the different opportunities to discuss prisoners' problems at different levels. Conflicts are part of life. Learning to handle them in different ways helps to prepare the prisoner for life in freedom. That conflicts can arise, is positive; that they are kept under control in different parts of the system (inmates, prison officers, management) is necessary. A situation in which all conflict is kept down, and no one is challenged, is not ideal.

A good example of this is the way the inmate newspaper *Die Posaune* discusses controversial topics, such as problems between the newspaper team and the in-house radio service *Die Trommel*; questions about the cleanliness of the courtyard; discussion of a particular attitude of a member of staff; criticism of the goods offered by the prison shop, and so on. The paper also describes events which passed successfully: pavement painting by some prisoners together with others in a local street, sporting events; it gives counsel on legal matters and discusses general issues in society. The paper appears every two months and is edited by the Governor.

In this connection it is worth mentioning the development of 'shared responsibility' schemes which have been obligatory for all prisons in Nordrhein-Westfalen since 1979. In free and secret elections all inmates can elect deputies to a council. All deputies are elected for two years and they have to be approved by the Governor. They meet once a week without supervision. They are not allowed to take up issues on behalf of a single prisoner, but can discuss with the management general questions concerning the life in the prison – local rules, food, leisure opportunities and so on. The climate of co-operation that this engenders allows big events such as an open air concert to happen without any problems.

A *Beirat* (advisory board) for the prison is appointed according to law, and six members drawn from politics, the Church, and unions meet regularly. They provide some overseeing of the work of the prison, represent the community; they allocate an hour a week to deal with prisoners' complaints.

### Education in prison

In 1989 a special occasion took place in Geldern: the first graduation of an inmate. A 28-year-old inmate had finished his university studies and graduated twice: in business and economics. Thirteen prisoners who study full time are located in a special department. An open university provides them with the necessary material for their studies by post. Since the installation of this study centre in 1983, some 36 prisoners have started full-time studies and have then been partially released or transferred to other prisons (open prisons or halfway houses). The most popular courses are economics, electrical engineering, mathematics and science-based subjects.

The open university material is not free and any student prisoner who has no funds available for such a course is entitled to seek help from the Ministry of Education, though any such grant is repayable by the prisoner. However, students who have sufficient funds and do not qualify for help from the Ministry of Education are subsidized by the Ministry of Justice – and these grants are not refundable. This curious bureaucratic anomaly is clearly unjust and is much resented.

### The staff

There are 180 prison officers at Geldern and, with office personnel, specialist services, teachers, etc., the overall total is about 250 staff.

Before being employed the potential prison officer has to take a test in writing, mathematics and psychology. Candidates are tested in Geldern Prison and about 60 per cent of them are refused after undertaking these tests. The prison officers wear a uniform, but no badge of rank. They do not carry weapons during the day, not even a stick or rubber truncheon, but are issued with a pistol for night duty. Firearms have been used just once since the prison was opened: warning shots when a prisoner tried to escape.

There is, as some of the officers noted, relatively strong competition for high-ranking posts. But overall, many officers still seemed to think that playing safe, being inconspicuous and making no mistakes was the most useful career plan. That meant being unwilling to look for promotion since, inevitably, it meant a higher risk. One of the seven shop stewards (two of whom work part time in order to free themselves for this union responsibility) confirmed this.

Many of the guards support the new targets of the prison administration, with its emphasis on resocialization, but there are also some who do not agree and a few who make no secret of their aversion towards the prisoners. To counterbalance this, a few are highly committed and even spend their leisure time on a voluntary basis if help is needed, for instance, to escort a prisoner on an outside visit.

Next to the prison buildings are some 42 flats (of from 94 to 148 sq.m) used as staff accommodation. The rent is low, but the neighbourhood around the prison suffers from being seen very negatively and there is a feeling that the prison, with its housing, has become little more than a ghetto.

## Summary

To determine whether a prison is performing a useful function one could ask three questions (arranged according to priority):

1  Is the physical and, as far as possible, the psychological integrity of the inmate secure? Is he safe in life and limb against threat from other inmates? Against excesses by the guards? Against torture? Are food and medical services adequate?
2  Is the dignity of the inmates protected as far as possible? This covers clothing, food, sanitation, the avoiding of arbitrary and petty rules, the availability of work, leisure facilities and visits from family and friends.
3  What does the prison offer for the further development of the inmate? This may be on the professional, personal, social and, if necessary, therapeutical level.

Problems can appear in all these three areas, whether from the legislative framework, the structure of the institution, or from the personal failings of those responsible for implementing the regime.

I thought that at Geldern the first and the second questions could be answered satisfactorily, so far as one can tell within a visit of a week. Concerning the third (opportunities for vocational development and training) the prison seems to be exemplary. Doubts do appear in connection with social work help and therapeutic assistance and these seem to derive from the organization of the institution. Because of the burden of reports and other administrative obligations, many of the psychologists and social workers are often considered as a part of the administrative system rather than as a confidential resource for the prisoners. Here is a fundamental problem: a penal system which on the one hand has to punish (by definition) and on the other hand wants to offer help – a help which only can be realized if mutual trust is established. The prisoner has to cope with the mixed message that the same institution is encouraging him with one hand while beating him with the other. This

166

tension surfaces openly in the role of the social work services which at the same time invite the inmate to trust and co-operate, even to the extent of revealing his weak points, yet exercise control and make judgements that directly affect his life. In discussions with prisoners psychological stress was identified as a problem and it seems to be inherent in the dual aims of the existing structure.

This is not to argue against a penal system which offers social and therapeutic help – on the contrary. It demonstrates the necessity of setting up a clear framework of conditions within which such help could be realized to the best advantage of both prisoner and staff. To this end one could envisage:

1   A gradual separation of administrative and therapeutic decisions (which needs mutual confidence and a sharing of power).
2   A development of the key position held by volunteers, who are automatically outside the administration. In Geldern about 20 per cent of the inmates are in regular contact with voluntary prison visitors who have their own legally defined status. They have their own opportunities for visits and are listened to by the administration in decisions about the respective inmates they know.

A special role is also held by two full-time priests in Geldern (one Catholic, one Lutheran) who both seem to have the confidence of the prisoners. A large room for church services, which is only used for religious purposes, is available to them and the atmosphere of trust and confidence which has grown up between them and the prisoners is obviously important. The priests also have a group of volunteers who help in a range of situations from craft work to debt counselling, and in the provision of help on release.

3   It is also worth considering whether therapeutic help could be provided which is not part of the prison administration. In two small units of the penal system in Nordrhein-Westfalen, Duren and Gelsenkirchen, this is already well established. Treatment may be paid for privately under this system, but may also be paid for by the prison authorities if recommended by the prison doctor. Any refusal of treatment ought not to be considered as automatically negative, nor should privileges depend on the 'progress' of any treatment plan.

A strategy based on these principles may create other problems. I realize that those working in the 'therapeutic' areas may not wish to be distanced from the means of making other decisions about the prisoner during his imprisonment. Separation of functions may be only a limited answer and if 'administration' and 'care' become too distanced or alienated it is unlikely to be of benefit to the prisoner. In Geldern Prison I saw this tension being played out in some of the staff roles, but there were also key individuals who managed to achieve a positive balance. One of the senior prison officers successfully combined a responsibility for security with the equally important role of empowering prisoners to take more responsibility for themselves. Nevertheless such individuals are rare. A gradual division of help and control, which keeps choices open for the prisoner, which values voluntary participation and which keeps re-integration in the community as its most important goal, remains the overall aim. Meanwhile, Geldern Prison is a step along the way.

## NOTE

1 This chapter was written before the recent reunification of East and West Germany.

# Chapter Ten

# THE TEXAS DEPARTMENT OF CORRECTIONS, USA

## *R.W. BURNHAM*

When John Howard died, 'Texas' was known only to a small number of Mexicans, American Indians and the occasional settler who had been thrown out of, or wandered away from, the established 'colonies' to the north and east. In historically accurate terms these settled states had ceased to be colonies fourteen years before Howard's death, but that probably did not much matter south and west of the Red River which forms the north-east boundary of what was then known as Tejas, or Tehas.

More settlers of North European stock gradually moved into present day East Texas at the end of the eighteenth century. A Spanish-dominated civilization had already spread north and east from Mexico. There was a continual potential for conflict between the two cultures, which eventually came to a dramatic crisis in the San Antonio area. The Spaniards had earlier established a chain of missions to 'civilize' the local population along the San Antonio River. Those beautiful mission buildings are still a major feature of Texas architectural history. One of them is called the Alamo and in 1836 became one of the shrines, not only of Texan history, but of the history of the United States. The Mexicans, under General Santa Anna, tried to retake some of the land that the newcomers had taken over. About 150 of those North European settlers chose to barricade themselves inside the Alamo Mission, turn it into a fortress, and to defy Santa Anna's army of around 5,000.

Instead of ignoring the Alamo and its small garrison, and pressing on to fight the main Texan army, Santa Anna decided to take the Alamo by storm. He succeeded, and all the resisters, including the famous Davy Crockett, died. Officially they are national heroes, but there are revisionist versions of history which make some, including Crockett, rather less heroic. The stand at the Alamo, however, did its job. Santa Anna lost so much time and so many men in a pyrrhic victory, for which he need never have fought in the first place, that when he finally met the full Texan force under General Sam Houston he was utterly defeated. Thereafter Texas became an independent country, with its own embassy in London, and ultimately a state of the Union.

That summary of early Texan history is included, not just for general interest, but to illustrate several factors which have always been characteristic of Texan culture, and so have influenced the history of prisons in the state. These factors are: conflict between cultures; a high proportion of displaced people and difficult arrivals; speed of social change; and perhaps above all, and certainly the most publicized, violence.

People from other cultures have compared living in the United States with living in a speeded-up film. That is perhaps strongest in California, where the feeling takes the form that the future has arrived before it was due. In Texas it may be described as the past constantly almost catching up with the future, leaving no stable present time. The Texas prison system may well have been one of the fastest expanding systems in recent history. That makes it very different from the prisons and bridewells about which Howard wrote. One of the themes running through *The State of the Prisons* is that with a few exceptions, neither numbers nor conditions of prisoners have changed very much since Howard first visited.

The ratio of prisoners, primarily adult males, to the population of Texas as a whole has usually been high, and higher than for most other American states. Prisons are big business in Texas. There can be few jurisdictions where the location of a major university programme was determined by the location of the oldest prison.

The prison population now stands at around 40,000, which was that of England and Wales prior to the 1980s increase, against a total state population of rather more than half that of England and Wales. In keeping with the tradition of doing things in a big way, the Texas authorities have always built large prisons. The Huntsville Unit, which is the original prison and is still in use, and known unofficially but universally as The Walls, accommodates close to 1,800. Huntsville was then a small agricultural town, and the population of the state probably a lot less than one million. Wandsworth and Pentonville, in London, with rather less capacity, were built at

170

about the same time to serve what was then the largest city in the world.

The Texas Department of Corrections (TDC) has continued to build big, and presumably Howard could not even have begun to imagine something like the Ellis I Unit, of over 2,000 beds. In Ellis I there are more people (300) on death row, than the total in any single prison that Howard saw. Death row is actually a prison within a prison. These details are given to emphasize the enormous difference of scale between any problem Howard dreamed of and the problems facing recent TDC directors.

The size of the state in the early days of the administration of justice led to a remarkable form of attempted commital to prison. According to one of my sources[1], it is the origin of the American term 'railroading', which has long been used as a slang term throughout the USA to mean compelling somebody to do something they do not want to do, and for which the legal or other administrative justification is marginal or dubious. In the late nineteenth century, the railroad network across the state was complete. The story goes that trains from distant towns had special coaches attached (or there were even dedicated special trains) to bring those sentenced to imprisonment for serious offences to Huntsville. Sometimes a resident of one of those towns was thought by one of his fellow citizens to be particularly obnoxious or dangerous, even though it was not possible to prove anything against him in law. A few of his fellow citizens would wait until the train was about to depart, nobble him and throw him on the train, slip the guards a few dollars and wave goodbye. When the train got to Huntsville, the prison authorities refused to admit him as there was no committal warrant. He therefore had the choice of making a new home somewhere or making his way back to a town about whose public feelings he could have no doubt, but knowing that if he did not change his ways the whole thing might happen again. It would be interesting to know the 'success rates' of such informal justice, but statistics are, understandably, lacking.

One long-standing feature of Texas prisons dating from the early times, and which occurred intermittently in many American prison administrations in the nineteenth and early twentieth centuries, was that of 'leasing out' prisons. Under that system an entrepreneur would pay the state to utilize the labour of the prisoners, normally by contracting them out to local farms. That frequently led to abuses and indeed sometimes to bizarre results. When in California, I was told that the site of San Quentin prison was determined by the fact that a leased prison hulk was inadequately tethered on the northeast side of San Francisco Bay. During a violent storm it broke away and drifted westwards until it hit land on the barren headland of San Quentin. It was easier to transport the guards there and order the convicts to start building their own new prison than to build new ships and take them back to Vallejo. As with the railroading story, I could find no confirmation, but the story of privatized prisons floundering without control or direction across San Francisco Bay, landing close to where Sir Francis Drake's memorial plaque was later found, may not be without a criminological moral.

The starting-point of that digression in time and place was that of leased prisons and the problems they increasingly raised for a socially responsible legislature. The development of a civil service style of correctional administration can serve as the starting-point for my main theme, a comparison of Howard's concerns with the changes, reforms and setbacks of prison administration in Texas since the Second World War. We could start with a review of his most famous chapters at the beginning of *The State of the Prisons*, especially the chapters entitled: 'General view of distress in prisons'; 'Bad customs in prisons'; 'Proposed improvements in the structure and management of prisons'. Those chapters summarize his main concerns, which are then illustrated in the narrative of the text with descriptions of individual institutions. As I discussed the history of changes in prisons with officials or ex-officials of TDC, or colleagues at the Criminal Justice Center, I came to think that the most logical order in which to look at the contemporary response to the questions that Howard raised was not the same as that which he followed in those chapters. Therefore I have taken the different topics in the order that my sources thought appropriate and provided references to at least some of the specific instances of those problems that Howard gave in his text.

The main question to which I return intermittently throughout this chapter, and with which it concludes, is one raised by implication in Howard's writings, but not addressed directly by him. That is the question of whether, in respect of prisons at least, people make the system what it is, or the system makes the people what they are. The history of TDC in the last decades has provided a remarkable case history of that problem, with examples of the arguments for and against each point of view. Such a review naturally includes questions of staffing quality, rules and regulations, classification, control of different kinds of abuses, prison employment and cleanliness, system comparison and where ultimate decision-making power is located.

The first step in the modernization of TDC was to appoint someone to improve what was widely acknowledged to be an unacceptable situation. Lee Simmons became director of TDC in 1930 with a reputation of being a hard but completely honest law enforcement officer. The 'straight cop' took over the 'bent screws', but lasted only four years; the explanation given being that he was a catcher, not a keeper. It seems a frequent theme in penal history that the two professions do not trust each other, at least as regards doing each other's job. After Simmons's departure in 1934 the situation deteriorated and escapes became a major problem, to such an extent that a most unusual political event occurred. Some ten years later the main plank in the platform of Beauford Jester as candidate for State Governor was prison reform, and he was elected on that campaign issue.

Modern Texas prison administration essentially dates from the steps Jester took to ensure that the prisons were run by an accountable board of people with a strong social conscience. Both the way he selected people and the status and accountability he gave them might have been suggested to him by John Howard.

Jester, his successor and the director they appointed, O.B. Ellis, all placed their central emphasis on the quality of staff, and the higher the grade, the more the quality counted. Ellis, according to his successor Beto, had two overriding overt concerns. The first was to enable the prison system to feed and clothe the prisoners through its own efforts. The second was with humane conditions in prisons, demonstrated above all by cleanliness. Howard would surely not have objected to either, although the idea of a department of corrections would have been very strange to him and the idea that it could act as a system to feed and clothe itself would presumably have seemed a desirable but unreal and irrelevant objective.

Ellis was succeeded by Beto, who has become a man of considerable controversy, both with supporters and detractors, in writings about the history of prisons. He was, and is, a strong advocate of the position that the right people make the system. One recent penal scholar, Di Julio, in his analysis of what is wrong with American prisons, regards Beto as a desirable role model (Di Julio 1987). A recent book by Martin and Ekland-Olson is much less positive (Martin and Ekland-Olson 1987). The reforms which have characterized the post-Ellis–Beto era derived from the actions of the believers in the supremacy of detailed legal guide-lines. The focus of the next sections is on those areas where the Ellis–Beto doctrine is seen at its best, and when it dominated TDC policy for twenty-five years. Ellis's obsessions, as noted, were self-sufficiency and cleanliness. One big advantage of self-sufficiency in food and clothing was that the demand on the public purse was much reduced. The state legislature was thereby able to be much more generous in capital grants for future building, and for improving the salaries of correctional officers.

The quality of staff was a recurring theme with Howard, and he placed emphasis on both appropriate remuneration (Howard 1792: 128, 129, 140, 158) and training (145, 173–4, 206, 222). In Howard's time, the main problem in respect of remuneration was that the gaoler was expected to generate his own income, by what often amounted to extortion from those in his charge or their family and friends. Howard was, therefore, in favour of a civil service system, although that concept was relatively new in the administration of Britain. Texas faced a similar problem throughout the 'leasing' period of the late nineteenth and early twentieth centuries. The standing of TDC officers as worthy of the wage of a respectable craftsman was not established until the Ellis era.

As an example, when Ellis died in 1962, a newly-recruited TDC guard received $256 per month with fringe benefits such as uniforms, and cannot have been highly regarded in a society which measures status by money. Both Ellis and Beto were as proud of their success in raising the salary and status of guards as they were of any other achievement. Howard would surely have approved of all that, but as so often in penal reform, the very advance of which the reformers were so proud led to an ironic and unforeseen development. An urgent need arose in the late 1970s and early 1980s to recruit many new prison guards. That crisis coincided with the beginning of an economic crisis, which saw south-east Texas in particular transformed within two years from one of the boom areas to one of the depressed areas of the USA.

For some decades, working for TDC had been a family tradition, and I met officials who were proud to be third generation prison men. In the towns around the main prisons, above all Huntsville, a culture of loyalty to TDC and a commitment to integrity and consistency had become established. The standards of humanity and gentility expected of guards, or shown towards prisoners, may not have been those of Alexander Paterson or the Howard League; but there *were* standards, which were informally learned and informally but forcefully demanded of the guards. In the early 1980s that tradition was broken by the need for new guards in combination with the growing unemployment rate.

It is widely believed both within TDC and by its critics that the relatively high pay levels established by the reforming directors of the 1950s and 1960s led to applications by, and the recruitment of, men who did not know of or subscribe to the old codes. The result was that the informal system of control by mutual understanding, with some mutual respect between prisoner and guard, was greatly weakened. The same good pay and conditions also coincided with the equal opportunities legislation which declared, in essence, that for all practical purposes there is no difference between the sexes. The recruitment of women therefore added to the degree of unsettling change experienced by the TDC system. Women guards supervise showering and conduct body searches on male death row. These guards seem unmoved, while many of the prisoners object; one can only speculate on what Howard's views would have been.

If there is a moral in the sequence of events as recounted above, it is that in penal reform there is always the potential for more influences to operate than those the planners have in mind.[2]

Howard's second concern with the quality of staff was with training, although he did not use that word. The improvement of the quality of work performed by criminal justice personnel through improved training has been much talked about and advocated since at least my own days as a trainee assistant governor almost thirty years ago, and probably well before that. Examination of what is entailed and what is expected have produced ambivalent conclusions, less clear than the raw conviction that training is a good thing: but overall the evidence is favourable. Beto has very definite ideas on this. Pre-service training is essential so that the staff know the rules and how to work in a disciplined system. In-service training is desirable only when it fulfils a felt need. Staff in a contemporary prison service or department of corrections come to believe that further training, or advanced training, or some other form of in-service training, is necessary if they are to become more 'professional'. One TDC guard remarked to me that it is like fibre in the diet. You don't miss it until somebody tells you that you need it; then you regard it as indispensable.

It is easy and almost certainly wrong to be cynical about in-service training. It is the only way yet devised to improve the professional morale and standing of a criminal justice agency, but, especially with lower ranking staff, it is extraordinarily difficult to demonstrate results.

Howard would have approved of the improvement in pay and conditions of service and greater emphasis on training but he might have been quite surprised at the eventual outcome of well-meaning initiatives. He would probably have been less confused or surprised at the implementation of some of his other priorities. One of the most fundamental of those was the importance of clearly-stated and widely publicized rules of conduct for both staff and prisoners (Howard 1792: 148, 152, 154, 166–9). Howard continually pointed out the arbitrariness of prison discipline, and the fact that such an evil was made possible primarily by the absence of formal, written, and published rules. He might have been surprised to know that before Ellis became director in 1950, the same was true in Texas. The importance which Ellis laid upon the drafting and promulgation of such rules is generally regarded as one of his major contributions to the civilizing of Texas prisons.

In addition to his open priorities discussed above, Ellis took office with two unpublished goals: the elimination of brutality and the elimination of petty theft. Both evils were perpetrated by both staff and prisoners. The abuse of prisoners by staff was a serious problem before Ellis took over. A major item in his creed was that prisons should be lawful. Each is a mini-society, and any society should be safe for all the members of that society. He considered that, since society had the right to lock people up, it had a corresponding obligation to ensure the safety of those locked up. Critics of the Ellis–Beto era contend that they traded off abuse by staff for abuse by inmates, in order to achieve a controlled and disciplined prison environment. That conflict of views has its fierce advocates on both sides, and I am neither well informed nor dispassionate enough to comment on it. From the presumed perspective of John Howard, the Ellis–Beto administrations overall emerge with credit, because they did insist on the publication of official rules, and that was a big breakthrough.

To refer once again to the unpredicted and possibly counter-productive side effects of the legal reform movement, the effect on the 'rules' question has been at most unfortunate in the eyes of many basic grade staff. In the earlier regime it was accepted that rules had to be general to some extent, and open to change to allow for adaptation to changing circumstances. After the courts inter-vened, the concern of the administration has to be not to leave itself open to any kind of charge of ignoring court rulings. To quote an anonymous source: 'The first rule in running prisons has always been to cover your arse. It is now the second, third and fourth rule as well.' In the more elegant terminology of another source, fossil-ization has set in and the push to drive out abuse has stifled the exercise of initiative.

One feature of prison rules as published in most administrations is that they require different provisions for different categories of prisoner. The concept of different categories requires the concept of classification, and that was one of Howard's preoccupations (Howard 1792: 127, 219). In his day, the main problem, to which he referred frequently, was the separation of adults from juveniles. In TDC institutions that separation was established and maintained many decades ago. It is apparently still the case that in some local, county gaols adults and juveniles are housed together, sometimes for periods of several weeks. The little evidence I could obtain suggested that the explanation was the usual one in criminal justice short-comings: a rising demand not met with increasing resources. Also the problem is increasingly severe the more local the gaol.

Howard might well have been impressed by the importance given to classification by TDC, despite the fact that it seems to be un-fashionable in western European administrations. Its associations with the treatment model, which has been so widely rejected, render it unacceptable. TDC has a Diagnostic Unit through which all newly sentenced prisoners pass. Beto describes diagnostic units as the Ford Edsells[3] of American corrections, although he does not claim to have invented the metaphor. He still defends their use on the grounds that 'For selfish reasons a prison administrator needs to know as much as he can about each prisoner, especially incoming prisoners.' The priority of the TDC classification scheme is to establish the needs of each individual prisoner. That diagnosis is not so much for therapeutic reasons as for administrative and management purposes.

The classification exercise provides another arena for the conflicting points of view as to the relative importance of good people as opposed to good systems. It is a debate which presumably would have appealed to Howard although his own views seem to have been that they are equally important. In the history of TDC since the Second World War, the struggle for supremacy of the contrasting viewpoints has been a *Leitmotiv*. The Ellis–Beto–Estelle (Estelle was Beto's successor) era was one in which the primacy of getting good people to do the important jobs was unquestioned. Since the Federal Court in the Eastern District of Texas, and subsequently the Fifth Circuit Federal Appellate Court seated in New Orleans intervened, the pendulum has swung and the emphasis has been on detailed rules to cover all contingencies, the implementation of which is far less dependent on the quality of individual personnel. One of Beto's constant themes is that classification is something which can be carried out properly only by staff who have both human insight in general and a specific knowledge of the prison system and the background of most of its clients. Classification by computer, howsoever sophisticated the algorithm, is not appropriate.

It is notable how classification is used as an instrument of control. That is clearly true and officially acknowledged in TDC. It could well become equally true in other systems as they grow to the size, complexity and pressures of TDC. In TDC the classification status of all prisoners is reviewed at least once a year, and sometimes as often as every ninety days. The decision resulting from that review can lead to a change of housing, work, and other living arrangements within an institution, or a change of institution. Not surprisingly it is regarded as an important and effective management tool. The visibility and accountability of the decision, or lack thereof, might have caused Howard some anxiety, but again he was not faced with proposing reforms for a prison system anything like as complex as TDC.

Another of Howard's themes was the damage done by mind-altering substances in prison (Howard 1792: 126, 135, 145, 159, 234). That rather ponderous phrase is used because in an unknown but not insignificant number of contemporary prisons the problem still exists, but the actual substance has changed. Howard protested against the use of alcohol in prisons, whereas the substances of abuse today in most administrations are drugs which are taken in small quantities and therefore can be smuggled in.

The sale of beer by the gaoler in late eighteenth-century Britain was apparently universal – Howard called it the 'tap' and seems to have regarded it as a necessary evil. His aim was to eliminate the importation of distilled spirits, for which his main rationale was the damage they did to health. That damage occurred in two ways. First was the direct effect of the dosage level on the general health of the prisoners. Second, and less obvious, was the diversion of resources from their 'proper' use of obtaining good food, to that of acquiring the drink.

The situation in TDC today is very different. Food is provided by the administration, while no alcohol is allowed, and it is difficult to smuggle it in. The main anxiety about diet which I heard expressed, at least by the administration, was that with the introduction of 'fast food' facilities, prisoners were showing the same dietary self-destructive tendencies as young teenagers traditionally have done. They prefer 'junk food' laden with additives, cholesterol and calories, but with very low nutrition value, to the less exciting but more nutritious food offered by the institution. Abuse of alcohol seems to be almost non-existent.

TDC officials believe that TDC is less badly affected than other prison administrations with respect to the smuggling in of narcotics and other drugs. Regular and thorough cell searches reveal syringes, hypodermic needles and other components of 'the works' only rarely. The drug problem is mostly limited to substances which produce recognizable behavioural patterns, normally some sort of muddled state or light-headedness. The explanation is either imported marijuana or the diversion of inhalants such as glue and paint stripper from the workshops. The sudden increase in staff from outside the prison culture may have resulted in there being more guards who themselves use marijuana in a limited recreational way, and who may not be averse to sharing a few joints with their charges. While senior officials recognize this as a problem requiring constant monitoring, the level of anxiety about it remains low, and it is not seen as the forerunner of a future threat.

While substance abuse has changed in both scope and nature, one of the other problems that vexed Howard (1792: 124, 128, 216) is still a major, and similar, difficulty for the TDC authorities. That is the need to provide employment for prisoners. In medieval Christendom the appropriate saying was 'The devil makes work for idle hands'. The idea was expressed in several languages. The version with which I was introduced to my housemaster role in the prison service by an experienced principal officer was 'One thing more difficult than a busy Borstal boy is an idle Borstal boy.' I believe that it is as close as we can ever come to a universal truth in the history of prisons – that lack of work for prisoners is the greatest cause of indiscipline, unrest and unhappiness among the prisoners. Idleness is feared there with good reason, and also to an obsessive degree, for, as has been observed, if men believe something to be true, it is true in its consequences.

One of Howard's obsessions was indeed that idleness and unemployment was the cause of many of the problems facing a prison administration. He would find an immediate echo in the different administrative offices of TDC in 1989. I have rarely if ever met a prison administrator, who does not subscribe to the doctrine that work for prisoners is the best training for life after release, and that it is also the best mechanism for running a humane and tidy prison. Neither have I come across much evidence to show that they are wrong.

One of the reasons advanced for the absence of meaningful work for prisoners in some administrations is that of the resentment of the outside world. The products of prisons are seen as taking over the market for the products of honest working men. That argument has been very forceful in some countries for the last three or four decades at least. Another of the ironies of penal reform is that it seems not to apply in Texas, one of the spiritual centres of capitalism. The weak tradition of trade unionism in Texas has been a major cause for the profession of the prison officer to develop in a very different way from in Europe. That same absence of union power has resulted in the absence of opposition to the marketing of TDC inmate products, either cotton measured in hundreds of tonnes or individually carved armadillos. Howard was strongly opposed to prison unemployment in the different circumstances with which he was familiar. He would have disapproved of it equally in contemporary western Europe and contemporary TDC, but he would have had to look for quite different explanations for its occurrence.

Agricultural hard labour, primarily the cultivation of cotton, had long been a prominent feature of TDC activity. The policy of Ellis, to feed and clothe the prison population from its own resources, has already been mentioned. Beto continued the policy but expanded the scope of inmate productivity to include building on a large scale. For many years new TDC plant, and some other related buildings, were built by prisoners; this included making the bricks. One of those buildings is the Criminal Justice Center at Sam Houston State University. The prisoners who built it left their own rather macabre memento by incorporating a hangman's noose into one of the rafters, with a nearby door leading into empty space and a four metre drop.

In the late 1970s the policy of building by prisoners was abandoned and the work put out to contract, as in most other jurisdictions. The usual explanation offered was the sudden need for more prisons. That need arose partly from the increasing number of convictions and sentences, and partly from the measures necessary to satisfy the newly-imposed court requirements. Prison labour may be efficient in terms of costs, but it is slow and requires a high degree of commitment of the staff at all levels. Organizing prisoner labour is, in fact, a very demanding job and one reason for the decline in its use was the effort it required of staff, including high level staff, to make it work properly.

Whatever the reason, the practice has now largely disappeared, and prisoner idleness is at a much higher level. As we can be sure that Howard would have approved of the constructive use of prisoners' time and energy and training in work habits, so we can probably also assume that he would have been disappointed in and disapproving of the latest trend.

One aspect of the TDC policy which seems to me to be both enlightened and enduring is the trouble which is taken to identify markets for work projects, particularly from the public sector, which again may sound surprising in capitalist Texas. For instance, one small independent public sector agency, the local school bus system, has made a contract for the maintenance of the buses, with another public sector agency, TDC. While the two agencies save each other money, they also keep out private business. The end result is curiously close to the situation which might be expected in a much more left-wing administration and with a high degree of efficiency and accountability.

The TDC administration is increasingly gearing its work programmes to the requirements of the State Purchasing Agency, as well as the expanding parts of the private sector. A successful field of trade training for prisoners is computer maintenance and utilization. Thus, while painting and decorating courses have rather faded because people do not want ex-prisoners inside their houses to decorate them, it is apparently much more acceptable to have an ex-prisoner in your house to repair your word-processor. At the time of writing, I understand that the computer training course has the highest rate of job placement for discharged prisoners of any vocational training programme in Texas prisons.

Along with unemployment and idleness, Howard hated dirt and over-crowding (Howard 1792: 135–7, 142–3, 151, 171–2). Beto is again a fellow spirit, for his recipe for the basic necessary conditions for a good prison, or any other total institution, consists of four absences:

1  Absence of idleness;
2  Absence of noise;
3  Absence of filth;
4  Absence of odour; the smell of disinfectant is a bad sign. It is a way of simulating cleanliness while actually covering up other odours of far less salubrious origin.

Cleanliness in TDC institutions has been a priority with the administration since Ellis's time at least. It was ensured primarily through the 'building tender' system: Some prisoners had a special status, half-recognized officially, derived from their job of 'tending the building' (hence the name), that is, to make sure that the cell blocks were kept clean. They were rather like the red-bands or trusties in British prisons. Their role included keeping an eye on the conduct of their fellows.

Perhaps in accordance with the less gentle side of Texas culture, 'keeping an eye on' was extended to forceful physical control, including arranging for 'necessary' beatings; and this abuse of power brought the 'building tender' system into disrepute. The issue became a central topic in the court rulings of recent years and the 'building tender' role was abolished. The cause of cleanliness has, however, not suffered because the function has been reintroduced, with strong safeguards. Certain prisoners, known as 'support service inmates', who have no authority, are responsible for cleanliness and some minor clerical work. But they are no longer the hard men who unofficially run the prison.

One cause of overcrowding in contemporary prisons, not only in Texas, has been the rise in the number of sentences of imprisonment imposed by the courts. Howard protested about overcrowding in conditions of a more or less stable prison population. The extent to which it could have been foreseen and thus pre-empted by a more alert administration, which tried to foresee coming trends, seems to be a matter of disagreement among prison administrators, critics and researchers in many jurisdictions. Beto is very proud, and I think justifiably so, that in the early 1960s he asked the Texas legislature at every session for a considerable amount of money to build for the future, and received it. Thus TDC was able to cope without overcrowding with the inexorable but still moderate increase in demand for capacity during the period 1955 to 1975. It is less sure that anyone in 1975 could have foreseen the dramatic increase in the demand for places in the ten years to follow. Likewise, if they had foreseen it, persuading political authorities to react on anything like the required scale and at the required speed would have been very difficult. I think it can be said fairly, that the management response, in a political climate moving steadily to the right, was always likely to be too little too late: but that observation applies in many jurisdictions other than Texas, and has the advantage of being based on hindsight.

The need for more prisons has appeared in many jurisdictions over the last fifteen years. If the overcrowding which Howard so decried is not to become worse, let alone be diminished, either courts must change their sentencing practices or more prisons must be built (Howard 1792: 170, 221, 224–5). There are, of course, the alternatives that people behave better and commit less crime; or that the police become less effective and catch fewer villains. But the former seems regrettably unlikely and the latter, over all, undesirable. More prisons entail more ground on which to build them. Public resistance to having a new prison near them is a common experience of administrations. It is known in Texas by the increasingly common term of NIMBYism – 'Not In My Back Yard'. Howard might well have experienced some kind of contemporary equivalent, and therefore, have been interested in the latest turn of events in Texas.

The effect on TDC of the change in the employment pattern of the state when the oil boom failed has already been mentioned. One discovery in the wake of that economic crisis by local communities is that prisons mean jobs, and a general boost to the local economy. I understand that more local communities have applied to TDC to be considered as 'host' towns for new prisons than TDC has plans to build them. The belief that unemployment increases both crime and the prison population independently as well as directly has long been held by criminologists of different persuasions. While the evidence for the validity of the hypothesis is much debated, the evidence against it is almost non-existent. It seems that in the case of Texas there is yet another irony of penal reform: unemployment increases the prison population, but also makes it possible to provide the new prisons for which the need has been created. Alas, there are no grounds, literally, for optimism on the part of European prison administrations from that example. There is still a lot of spare or marginally used land in Texas.

The increasing control of TDC by the Texas courts has been referred to several times already. The crucial case, something of a watershed in Texas prison history, was *Ruiz* v. *Estelle*. It was first brought in 1972, but its implications became clear only several years later. The case was so complicated that it has already generated at least two books (Crouch and Marquart 1989, Martin and Ekland-Olson 1987) and more might be on the way. It would be appropriate here simply to give a brief outline of events, and then limit any review to the ways in which it is relevant to John Howard and his cause.

There is a much stronger tradition in American society than in British of rectifying perceived private wrongs by means of litigation. When the defendant is a public body of some kind, the chief executive officer is quite often named in the law suit. When *Ruiz* v. *Estelle* appeared in the court lists in front of Federal Judge Justice, it seemed a fairly run-of-the-mill event, for several prisoners had filed suits before. Ruiz sued TDC for violations of his rights under the first, fourth and eighth amendments to the Constitution of the United States.

The state decided to defend the charges. Opinion in Texas prison circles, with hindsight, seems to be that TDC should simply have admitted that various provisions for prisoners were unsatisfactory and inadequate. It could then have pleaded force of circumstances and lack of resources, not as a defence but as an excuse. As it was Judge Justice had to rule against it with all the authority of the Supreme Court of Texas. Instead of a telling-off, with time to put

184

things right, TDC found itself under a much more strict court order with which it could not negotiate and which gave it little flexibility. Through some clever legal work on behalf of other prisoners bringing litigation, various other cases were incorporated into the Ruiz decision.

The results of the decision are still making themselves felt. As far at I could judge it, the general feeling among the present day staff is that there have been some gains to both the prisoners and the system, and some losses, but the gains have been bought dearly and slowly and the losses may be irreversible. The main gains are a better staff–inmate ratio, and a greater focus on programmes for inmate recreation and on putting the prisoners' time to better use, apart from compulsory work. The main losses have been in the relations between staff and the prisoners. Most prison reformers, including Howard, have emphasized that any rehabilitative effect which prison may have will derive primarily from the quality of the relationship built up between a respected member of staff and an individual prisoner. It seems that on human relationships within the prison the long-term effects of the Ruiz decision have been mostly negative.

I should emphasize that the summary account given above is not at all official, and has no claim to comprehensiveness or objectivity. I have simply reported the reactions of various past and present TDC officials with whom I spoke, and of some of my colleagues on the faculty of the Criminal Justice Center. Those interested in an authoritative and detailed account are referred to the books cited, but are also advised that the whole issue is one on which sides have been taken, and disinterested views are rare.

The significance of the Ruiz case and its aftermath for any analysis of the significance of the work of John Howard lies within the example it gives of a certain approach to penal reform. To pick up on an earlier theme, there are two main traditions in penal reform. The first, stretching from Howard through Paterson to Ellis and Beto, is, as observed, that the crucial step is to find the right people, particularly for the top jobs. With good men, goodness will trickle down, and discretion will be wisely used to allow flexibility and fairness to coexist, even in a prison. The critics of that view ask what happens if, or indeed when, goodness fails to trickle down far enough or fast enough. They tend to answer by pointing to such undesirable developments as the 'building tender' system.

The alternative to the 'good men' model is the 'good rules' or good system model. The unfolding of the implications of the Ruiz decision illustrate the weaknesses of that approach. Perhaps the most important of these is the difficulty of long-term planning, because it is impossible to predict what events will be brought before the courts, and how the courts will decide upon them. There is a permanent element of uncertainty built into the situation, which undermines the willingness of administrators to make long-range commitments or plan for flexibility. It tends to encourage any tendency to the suppression of initiative, and to foster cautious conservatism, perhaps to the point of atrophy.

I have represented both approaches simplistically, to draw out the contrast specifically because it seems that Howard favoured both approaches, but did not have the experience of both to see the contradictory implications. For instance, 'I am persuaded that a good gaoler can more easily manage his prisoners by humane attention than by severity and heavy irons' (Howard 1792: 145) (writing about Maidstone County Gaol). Four pages later, when writing about Aylesbury Bridewell, he said, 'the prisoners here wished that the magistrates had made rules also for them' (Howard 1792: 149). (The 'also' refers to the fact that the magistrates had made rules for the county gaol close by.) It is possible to infer from these passages and others in *The State of the Prisons* that Howard believed in both the good man theory, and in control by the courts. On the local scale in which he was operating, the two approaches may indeed have been symbiotic. My experience in Texas and with other large contemporary prison systems leads me to wonder whether in future the best we can hope for is to obtain some kind of a mix of the two, and avoid the worse features of each.

## ACKNOWLEDGEMENT

I wrote this chapter as the George J. Beto Chair Professor at the Criminal Justice Center, Sam Houston State University, Huntsville, Texas for the spring of 1989. I wish to record my gratitude to the Dean and Faculty of the Center for that opportunity, and for my professionally valuable time in Huntsville. George Beto, now in semi-retirement but still teaching at the Center, is one of the main actors in the story. He was also my main source of information, and a personal friend; he could be considered the co-author of this chapter. In so far as it comments extensively on his main life work, usually but not always positively, it seems more appropriate that his contribution, while fully acknowledged, should be classified as 'informal'. He also put me in touch with the other two main Texas Department of Corrections (TDC) or academic sources whose knowledge I have used. I should mention in particular Associate Warden J. Lampert of TDC, and my faculty colleagues at the Criminal Justice Center.

## NOTES

1 Dr Wayland Pilcher, Professor of Criminal Justice, Sam Houston State University.
2 The Texas (and presumably elsewhere in the USA) version of Murphy's Law is 'There is always one more son-of-a-bitch than you reckoned on.'
3 A model of car introduced by Ford Motor Company in the 1950s with much fanfare, and a subsequent record of being unbought by the public. The term has become synonymous for many Americans with the 'well-intentioned but ill-thought-out' product.

## REFERENCES

Crouch, B.M. and Marquart, J.W. (1989) *An Appeal to Justice: Litigated Reform of Texas Prisons*, Austin, Texas: University of Texas Press.
Di Julio, J.J. (1987) *Governing Prisons: a Comparative Study of Correctional Management*, New York: The Free Press.
Howard, J. (1792) *The State of the Prisons in England and Wales* (facsimile of 4th edn), vol. 2.
Martin, S. J. and Ekland-Olson, S. (1987) *Texas Prisons: The Walls Come Tumbling Down*, Austin, Texas: The Texas Monthly Press.

# JOHN HOWARD

*A biographical note*

*DICK WHITFIELD*

The bi-centenary of the death of John Howard in 1990 has given rise to a number of commemorative events in varying parts of the world, of which this book is one. That in itself is some indication of the influence his life and work still bring to bear – and, perhaps, an equal indication of the lack of progress which makes it still necessary. His book, *The State of the Prisons*, a uniquely systematic description of conditions in British and European prisons in the last part of the eighteenth century, is an astonishing monument.

In the course of this odyssey, and at a time when travel was usually uncomfortable and often dangerous, he travelled nearly eighty thousand kilometres on horseback and spent some £30,000 of his own money in his determination to improve prison conditions; he entered prisons in disguise in defiance of governments who feared the power of his pen; was captured by pirates; quelled a riot single handed and more than earned John Wesley's tribute to him as 'one of the greatest men in Europe'.

This account of his life and work is included as a reminder of how one man, from unremarkable beginnings, could have such a remarkable impact in a sphere characterized only by indifference. Sir Walter Scott later wrote, 'Without courage, there cannot be truth; and without truth there can be no other virtue.' Howard had the courage to put his conviction into practice. He saw the pains of imprisonment and used truth as the agent of change, not from any intellectual theory or ideology but through a sense of compassion for other human beings. His own story provides a fitting conclusion for this book.

Reliable facts about John Howard's early life are hard to come by; his birth, on 2 September 1726, is variously located at Enfield in

Middlesex and Hackney in East London. What follows are the most reliable facts which his early biographies (John Aiken, 1792 and James Baldwin Brown, 1823) provided and which have subsequently been checked and accepted, as far as possible, from his own works and from later accounts.

The Howard family background was solid, middle class and prosperous. Howard's father was a London merchant and small businessman who specialized in upholstery and carpets and the family also owned a small farm at Cardington in Bedfordshire, some 80 km north of London.

John's formal education began at the age of six, when he was sent to the school of a Mr Worsley in Hertford. It continued at Mr John Eames's Moorfields Dissenting Academy in London, but it seems that young Howard did not take readily to formal learning and to the end of his life he remained only indifferently literate. His published works were normally edited by a friend before being submitted for printing. He did not proceed to university in his seventeenth year but was instead apprenticed for £630 to the London wholesale grocery firm of Newnham and Shipley, in Watling Street. It was a large indenture payment and coming, as it did, soon after his father's death in March 1743, was probably intended to secure a profitable mercantile future for him. It was certainly a comfortable start; his allowance permitted him an apartment, a body servant and two horses. However, he got out of the commitment and at the age of 20 embarked on the first of many journeys to Europe. It seems to have been an independent version of the Grand Tour and was an early indication of the restless urge to travel which he never lost. Howard later said that 'my continuing long . . . in any place lowers my spirits', and he tried to cure what was described as 'a species of nervous fever and of a general weakness of the whole system' by visiting resorts such as Bristol Hot Wells. It was a debilitating time and he felt he survived it for two reasons – a 'rigorous regime', which included a vegetarian diet, and the devoted nursing of his widowed landlady, Sarah Lordore (or Lardeau) at his lodgings in Stoke Newington.

They married on 15 October 1753, but it proved to be a short-lived union for she died only two years later. Shortly afterwards Howard left Stoke Newington and moved back to central London, to St Pauls Churchyard, where he owned several houses in the neighbourhood. His reaction to his new situation was perhaps predictable – he decided to travel again, both for interest and to reflect on his own future. Early in 1757 he sailed for Portugal, intending to view the results of Lisbon's great earthquake but his ship, the *Hanover*, was captured by a French privateer and passengers and crew were all taken prisoner and held in France, first at Brest and then at Morlaix.

John Howard became the spokesman for the group and was eventually released on parole to return to England to negotiate the exchange and release of his fellow-prisoners – a task he successfully accomplished. There followed a rather more conventional period where his activities seem to have differed little from the other young gentlemen of his day; he studied scientific works on medicine and the natural sciences and pursued a particular interest in taking thermometer readings under varying conditions, including some from the craters of Italian volcanoes. In 1756 he was elected a Fellow of the Royal Society and he continued his temperature recordings, contributing to its journal on three occasions.

His second marriage was more conventional. His bride Henrietta Leeds was a distant cousin, then aged 32. She came from an eminent legal family and the wedding took place at Croxton, Cambridgeshire, where her family had a home, on 2 May 1758. Perhaps it was this legal background which encouraged Howard to enter into a formal agreement with Henrietta which laid down that 'to prevent altercations about those little matters which he had observed to be the chief grounds of uneasiness in families – he should *always* decide'. How much Henrietta kept to the terms of the arrangement we do not know. The couple returned to the Howard estate at Cardington in Bedfordshire at first but moved for a time to Lymington on the Hampshire coast later, for the sake of her health. Henrietta's frail constitution could not withstand the rigours of childbirth, however, and after seven years of marriage she died soon after giving birth to their son, John.

The infant John was to become the disappointment of his father's life. Little is known for certain about his early upbringing or education although we do know that John Howard was criticized for both neglecting him (because of his many absences) and for imposing an unduly repressive regime when he was at home. John, Junior, went to school at Nottingham and – briefly – to the University of Edinburgh. It was at St John's College, Cambridge, which he entered in the summer of 1784 that matters really came to a head, however. He was dismissed for gross misconduct, which seems to have centred on drug taking and homosexual activities. The following year, while Howard was on a tour of prisons in Europe which was to last 14 months, his son became psychotic. He was committed to a private asylum in Leicester, where he remained until his death in 1799.

The seven years of his second marriage were a stable and satisfying period for Howard and the time when he largely established himself as a country gentleman. He became a model landlord, a horticulturalist (he won a gold medal from the Royal Society for some successful experiments with a variety of potatoes) and he began to put into practice some of the notions of public service which he felt appropriate to his station in life. He became the road supervisor for his parish and oversaw the construction of a unique causeway road to Cardington; the model cottages on his estate for industrious and sober tenants were much admired and his considerable energy and interest in education were put to good use locally.

Cardington parish at that time was a small agricultural community of some 900 people, mostly concentrated in Cardington village or the three surrounding hamlets. Most were labourers and were tenants of either Howard or the lord of the manor, Samuel Whitbread. Howard, who was becoming a country gentleman with some town property (as opposed to his father, who would have seen himself as a London merchant with a country house), set about enlarging and redecorating his 'country seat'. But it was the ability to become a socially responsible landlord which gave him most satisfaction. Some two dozen of his tenants were re-housed in new brick, thatched houses, each with its own garden, and he was careful to look after their employment, health and education needs in return for steady work, church attendance and sober habits. By 1782 he was paying for 16 boys and 7 girls aged 4 to 11 to attend the local school, and contributing money to build the local workhouse.

After his wife died, Howard again took to travelling; but Cardington was now firmly established as his base and he had sufficient esteem in the eyes of his neighbours to be appointed High Sheriff of Bedforshire in 1773. So began the chain of events which ensured that his name remains so widely known, two centuries later, because with the title of High Sheriff came the responsibility for the county gaol.

Most High Sheriffs regarded this responsibility as purely nominal, impinging rarely and normally only when a new gaoler had to be found. The gaoler was appointed, made his living as best as he could from bribes, favours, anxious relatives and profits from the already meagre food allocation – and was allowed to get on with it. Yet everyone knew of the abuses which had grown, flourished and even became institutionalized in this *laissez-faire* prison system. There were probably around 5,000 prisoners on any one day in England at that time, spread between almost 250 gaols, prisons and houses of detention. Up to 500 were in the largest establishment, Kings Bush Prison in London, but most were in small town and provincial lock-ups in which only a handful of prisoners were kept. Many of the smaller gaols formed the rear of public houses with the publican doubling his duties with that of gaoler. To avoid the window tax many were either devoid or severely deficient in natural light.

That, in many ways, was the least of the problems. Among the customs prevalent in gaols were those such as garnish, fotting or chummage, which all gave the same message to newcomers – 'pay or strip'. Those having no money were forced to give up their clothes and sleep on the bare floor, often with fatal results. Prisoners were loaded with irons, which made walking and sleeping painful or near impossible; gaolers would, of course, grant dispensation for those who could pay sufficient to have them removed. Howard, writing in 1775, notes:

> Convicts were generally robust young men who had been accustomed to free diet, tolerable lodgings and rigorous exercise. On entering Hereford prison they were ironed: thrust into close, offensive dungeons, some of them without straw or bedding and remained two thirds of the 24 hours utterly inactive. Ely Gaol was the property of the Bishop and because of the insecurity of the old prison the gaoler chained the victims down on their backs on the floor, across which were several iron bars, with an iron collar with spikes about their necks and a heavy iron bar over their legs.

Worst of all were the arbitrarily imposed 'delivery' or discharge fees which often meant innocent people spending substantial periods in prison (having been found not guilty) until hard-pressed relatives raised the necessary cash for release and the gaoler was prepared to let them go. The net result of a system which mixed young and old, debtors and criminals, men and women, first offenders and old lags indiscriminately was, inevitably, that prisoners were exploited, brutalized and deprived of even the few rights that the law allowed them. In turn, prisoners survived by exploiting and brutalizing their weaker fellows, thereby reinforcing all the anti-social tendencies which had driven them there.

Howard probably knew some of this, even if vaguely, long before he became High Sheriff. Most of his contemporaries would have shrugged their shoulders and let it remain as part of the natural order of things. Instead, Howard visited Bedford Gaol and, shocked by what he saw, determined to do something about it. He was particularly disturbed by the practice of detaining prisoners until their 'board and lodging' fees had been paid to the gaoler and wondered why a salary could not be paid to avoid the corruption inherent in the fee system. It was typical of the thoroughness of his approach that he immediately decided to visit sixteen gaols in near-by counties so that he could gauge the extent of the evil, look for alternative solutions and make out a proper case for reform.

It was a shocking experience and to the abuses of the gaolers was added the deadly lottery of gaol fever and smallpox, pneumonia and diphtheria. Of gaol fever, which we now know as typhus, Howard later wrote:

> From my own observations I was fully convinced that many more were destroyed by it than were put to death by all the executions in the kingdom. But the mischief is not confined to prisons – multitudes catch the distemper by going to their relatives and acquaintances in the gaols; many others from prisoners discharged; and not a few in the courts of judicature . . . . Even if no mercy were due to the prisoners, the gaol distemper is a national concern of no small importance.

This was no understatement: the problem went back at least a century to the 'Black Assize' at Oxford where 'all who were present died in 40 hours; the Lord Chief Baron, the Sheriff and about 300 more' (Pettifer 1939: 17). In 1730, at the Somerset Assizes, the deadly fever similarly affected judges, barristers' clerks and prisoners until several hundred were dead, and in 1750 there was a virulent outbreak at the Old Bailey. Among those present at the trials, the Lord Mayor, two judges, an alderman, an under-sheriff and fifty others, from prisoners to jury-men, all perished.

Howard subscribed to the contemporary theory that the disease was transmitted by vapours (it is, in fact, caught by man through the bites of body lice) and well knew how much at risk he put himself each time he entered the noxious cells. A handkerchief drenched in vinegar was often all that could be done but he added, 'I seldom enter an hospital or prison before breakfast; in an offensive room I avoid drawing my breath deeply; and on my return sometimes wash my mouth and hands.'

The emphasis in Howard's books on simple hygiene, on ventilation, sanitation and the whitewashing of interior walls is hardly surprising. Some biographers have commented on the excessive detail in which he considers every part of the physical aspects of imprisonment – the air supply and water and sewage arrangements, bathing, sterilization of verminous clothing, beds, bedding and diet. Yet Howard saw, all too often, that the effect of a prison sentence might be health so broken that the ex-prisoner was unemployable.

There were other issues, too. 'In some gaols you see', wrote Howard, 'boys of twelve or fourteen eagerly listening to the stories told by practised and experienced criminals, of their adventures, successes, stratagems and escapes.' Howard not only proposed segregation by sex and of hardened felons from the younger, more tractable ones; he proposed day rooms, useful work and single cells. These were not the ideals of a humane but impracticable observer – Howard pursued the problem with unusual rigour and much to the amazement of many of his friends.

Within a year he had given detailed and authoritative evidence to the House of Commons and been instrumental in the passage of two bills which abolished gaolers' fees and enabled counties to pay for a proper service; which allowed discharged defendants to be set at liberty in open court; and which not only improved sanitation and health arrangements but made it obligatory for justices to have a concern for the health of prisoners. It was a startling achievement in such a short time. Howard was not only thanked by Parliament for his humanity and zeal; he even had copies of the Act printed at his own expense and distributed to all gaol keepers.

In doing so, he probably realized how difficult the process of change was likely to be. The new regulations were, at first, systematically evaded by all those with vested interests and he recognized that to pursue the path he had begun he was going to have to reinforce the need for change again and again. During 1775 he continued prison visiting in England and expanded his enquiries to the continent. Two years later his most famous work, *The State of the Prisons in England and Wales, with preliminary observations and an account of some foreign prisons,* was published. It provides an extra-ordinarily careful and detailed picture and records – factually and unemotionally – the abuses which characterized the whole system.

Above all, he made sensible, measured recommendations for improvement. As noted earlier, many of these concerned the design, construction and physical requirements, but he had an equal amount to say about the administrative aspects. Pressing for the abolition of the pernicious fee system had been an obvious target but he also pressed for liquor taps to be banned and the sale of drink to inmates to be closely regulated; for the gaolers to be resident at the gaol instead of offering only minimal supervision if they lived away from it; for the provision of chaplains and doctors and the detailing and publishing of prison rules and regulations. He also advocated the appointment of prison inspectors and made it clear that he expected them to be as thorough as he himself had been, probing every corner and speaking with every prisoner.

His great virtue was that he did not rely on a single visit, but frequently returned after a period of years and was able to comment on progress – or lack of it – and the way in which new legislation was being implemented. He remained an extraordinarily influential one-man pressure group and continued to give evidence on prison conditions to the House of Commons.

Howard had to deal with criticism, too. The usual views were advanced – that he would make prison too 'soft' and too attractive; that treating lawbreakers well would encourage more crime and that prisoners were undeserving and irredeemable, anyway. He met these full on. He was adamant that his proposals would not destroy the deterrent value of prisons; on the contrary, the prohibition of all 'riotous amusement' would ensure that they were 'sufficiently irksome and disagreeable, especially to the idle and profligate'. His statement on the handling of prisoners is worth quoting in full:

The notion that convicts are ungovernable is certainly erroneous. There is a mode of managing some of the most desperate, with ease to yourself, and advantage to them. Many of them are shrewd and sensible; manage them with calmness, yet with steadiness; show them that you have humanity, that you aim to make them useful members of society; let them see and hear the rules and orders of the prison, and be convinced that they are not de-frauded in their provisions and clothes by contractors or gaolers;

when they are sick, let them be treated with tenderness. Such conduct would prevent mutiny in prisons and attempts to escape; which I am fully persuaded are often owing to prisoners being made desperate, by the inhumanity and ill-usage of their keepers.

Howard practised what he preached. During one of his European tours he arrived at a prison in the Savoy where a full-scale riot was in progress and two warders had already been killed. Despite vehement advice to stay out, he insisted on entering the prison on his own, where the calmness and mildness of his approach enabled negotiations to begin. He listened to grievances, gave some measured advice of his own and enabled a savage dispute to be settled by both sides with dignity.

Howard's reputation in Europe was, if anything, more influential than at home. He visited prisons in France, Holland, Austria, Prussia, Denmark, Sweden and Russia – but it took time to establish his authority and certainly his relationships with administrators and staff were often initially imbued with deep suspicion or outright opposition.

He had to use subterfuge and bluff on many occasions, and was not above resorting to disguise. He sometimes smuggled in a small set of balance scales in order to be able to weigh the prisoners' rations when he discovered how much the system was open to abuse; he was also quite capable of openly exploiting the rules, if needed. Refused admission to French prisons, he discovered an ancient regulation which permitted entry to those giving alms to the prisoners, so promptly made use of it. In fact, only three significant prisons remained unvisited by Howard: the Bastille, the Prison of the Inquisition in Rome and the Doge's Prison in Venice. Elsewhere, his reputation and his persistence opened all gates, even in Tsarist Russia.

*The State of the Prisons* went through four editions as Howard's travels and experience grew and a second book, *An Account of the Principal Lazarettos in Europe*, reflected his later interest in military hospitals, lazarettos for the sick, and ways of combating the plague. He was very much involved in the process of publication as this account makes clear:

Lodgings were taken near to the printers and no journeyman printer could have worked harder than Howard himself did. He rose every morning at two, and worked at the correction of proofs till seven, when he breakfasted. Punctually at eight he repaired to the printing-office and remained there until the workmen went to dinner at one, when he returned to his lodgings and, putting some bread and raisins, or other dried fruit in his pocket, generally took a walk in the outskirts of the town during their absence, eating, as he walked along, his hermit fare, which, with a glass of water on his return, was the only dinner he took . . . .

When he had returned to the printing-office, he generally remained there until the men left work and then repaired to Mr. Aiken's house, to go through with him any sheets which might have been composed during the day; or, if there were nothing on which he wished to consult him, would spend an hour with some other friend, or return to his lodgings, where he took his tea or coffee, in lieu of supper; and at his usual hour retired to bed.

(Gibson 1901)

It was a spartan regime. Howard himself told an interviewer in 1789 that his daily diet consisted of 'two penny rolls with butter or sweetmeats, one pint of milk, five or six cups of green tea and at bedtime a roasted apple'. Although tolerant of the religious beliefs of others, his belief in the work ethic and his intolerance of alcohol made him insist on a stern regime for others. There is a record of a severe lecture he delivered to Capuchin monks in Prague whom he found were living far more expansively than his own abstemious style would permit.

The cost of his travels and his books (many of which were distributed free or sold at a subsidized price) was heavy. His annual income when he died was £496, which may seem a fortune compared with the £20 earned annually by a farm labourer but was modest compared with that of most country gentlemen. His son's incarceration at the Belle Grove Asylum cost £200 per year and by the 1780s he was having to dispose of properties in London and Middlesex in order to pay for his European journeys. For the final tour he even borrowed £1,000, interest free, from his friend and neighbour, Samuel Whitbread. In all, between 1773 and 1790, he is reckoned to have spent £30,000 of his own money and to have devoted a third of his time to his crusade to record and improve prison conditions. This short, thin, sallow man went quietly and doggedly about his business; observant, methodical, fired by religious enthusiasm and a passionate conviction until his message was too insistent to be denied. He believed in self-reformation, a voluntary rather than a coercive process, and wrote:

> Our present laws are certainly too sanguinary, and are therefore ill executed; which last circumstance, by encouraging offenders to hope that they may escape punishment, even after conviction, greatly tends to increase the number of crimes. Yet many are brought to a premature end, who might have been made useful to the state.
>
> I the more earnestly embarked in the scheme of erecting penitentiary-houses from seeing cartloads of our fellow creatures carried to execution; [many of whom] I was fully persuaded might, by regular, steady discipline in a penitentiary house have been rendered useful members of society; and above all from the pleasing hope that such a plan might be the means of promoting salvation of some individuals – of which, every instance is, according to the unerring word of truth, a more important object than the gaining of the whole world.

Howard saw many of the practices he wanted to introduce already being used in Europe. In Holland, he reported that 'there are so many rooms, that each prisoner is kept separate'; in Switzerland felons had a room to themselves 'that they might not tutor one another'. He added:

> to the penitentiary-houses I should wish that *none* but old, hardened offenders, and those who have . . . forfeited their lives by robbery, housebreaking and similar crimes, should be committed; or, in short those criminals who are to be confined for a long term, or for life.

Holland was the country that impressed him most:

> I leave this country with regret as it affords a large field for information on the important subject I have in view. I know not which to admire most – the neatness and cleanliness appearing in prisons, the industry and regular conduct of the prisoners, or the humanity and attention of the magistrates and regents.

Howard's influence as a kind of unofficial gadfly and inspector of prisons was significant; his parliamentary and legislative contribution more so, although in retrospect there seem to have been missed opportunities and errors. He was at least partly associated with the decision to introduce 'hard labour' into prisons, but far from providing regular, steady discipline and useful work it became drudgery of the hardest and most servile kind, a hated example of the additional pains of imprisonment. And he advised Parliament, when a House of Commons committee was enquiring into the provisional continuance of the prison hulks system in 1778, that conditions had improved since his earlier criticisms and that he would support continued use of the hulks until transportation could be resumed. Considering the wretchedness for which these floating prisons later became infamous it was an unhappy endorsement and one can only assume that his short-term view of a particular problem was allowed to obscure his longer term aims.

Perhaps the best judgement comes from one of his contemporaries, Burke, in a speech at Bristol:

> he visited all Europe – not to survey the sumptousness of palaces or the stateliness of temples; but to dive into the depths of dungeons . . . to survey the mansions of sorrow and pain, to take the gauge and dimensions of misery, depression and contempt; to remember the forgotten, to attend to the neglected, to visit the forsaken and to compare and collate the distresses of all men in all countries. His plan is original; it is as full of genius as it is of humanity. It was a voyage of discovery, a circumnavigation of charity. Already the benefit of his labour is felt more or less in every country. I hope he will anticipate his final reward by seeing all its effects fully realized in his own.
>
> (Stoughton 1884)

Apart from prisons, Howard's abiding interest was in the prevention and treatment of contagious diseases and his later visits to hospitals and lazarettos (port-side institutions where suspect goods and personnel could be quarantined) were just as important to him as his continuing battle against gaol fever. He had no formal medical training but had physicians as close friends, carried a medical kit on his travels and actually prescribed treatment on occasions. His work in this area won him honorary membership of the London Medical Society.

Perhaps inevitably, he eventually contracted typhus at Kherson, in the Crimea, in January 1790 and was dead within a few days. He was touring Russia and Eastern Europe in search of new material and had already accumulated notes on forty-one prisons and hospitals.

Such was his reputation that 2,000 people attended his funeral in Russia and one of the first statues in St Paul's Cathedral in London was not of a sovereign, statesman or saint – but a simple, teetotal, vegetarian traveller who, as the inscription notes:

> Had the fortune to be honoured whilst living
>   In the manner which his virtues deserved;
>   He received the thanks
> Of both houses of the British and Irish parliaments
> For his eminent services rendered to his country
>   And to mankind.
> Our national prisons and hospitals,
> Improved upon the suggestions of his Wisdom
> Bear testimony to the solidity of his judgement
> And to the estimation in which he was held
> In every part of the Civilised World
> Which he traversed to reduce the sum of
>   Human Misery.

All of this is a world removed from Howard's own wishes. 'Lay me quietly in the earth', he requested, '. . . no monument to mark where I am laid. Place a sundial over my grave and let me be forgotten.'

His work has ensured a different fate.


## BIBLIOGRAPHY

Howard's own major work, *The State of the Prisons in England and Wales*, was published in Warrington, Lancashire, by William Eyres in 1777, 1780 and 1784 and his *Account of the Principal Lazarettos in Europe* by the same publisher in 1789. A second edition of the latter work was published posthumously in London in 1791, as was a fourth edition of *The State of the Prisons* a year later. Subsequent editions have included the famous Everyman's edition (J.M. Dent, London, 1929) and the splendid Patterson, Smith reprint of the 2nd edn (Montclair, New Jersey, 1973, 2 vols), from which quotations are made in this chapter.

Books on Howard and his work are varied and considerable in number. A full bibliography by Leona Baumgarter was published by the Johns Hopkins Press (Baltimore, 1939) under the title: *John Howard (1726–1790), Hospital and Prison Reformer: A Bibliography.*

Some important works on Howard are:

Aiken, Dr J. (1792) *A view of the character and public services of the late John Howard*, London: J. Johnson.

Brown, J.B. (1823) *Memoirs of the Public and Private Life of John Howard, the Philanthropist*, London: Underwood.

Dixon, H. (1849) *John Howard and the Prison World of Europe*, London: Jackson & Walford.

Freeman, J. (ed.) (1978) *Prisons Past and Future*, London: Heinemann.

Gibson, C.S. (1901) *John Howard*, London: Methuen & Co.

Howard, D.L. (1958) *John Howard: Prison Reformer*, London: Christopher Johnson.

Pettifer, E.W. (1939) *Punishments of Former Days*, Bradford: Cleggs.

Southwood, M. (1958) *John Howard: Prison Reformer*, London: Independent Press.

Stoughton, J. (1884) *Howard the Philanthropist and his Friends*, London.

# NAME INDEX

Alexander, Daniel 13–14
Anderson, Erik 7

Barse, Sheela 51
Baxi, U. 35, 53 n.10
Beto, G.J. 173–4, 176–8, 181–3, 185
Bhagwati, Justice 35–6, 51
Borge, Tomas 126, 127
Breytenbach, Breyten 85 n.3
Brockway, Fenner 3–4
Brydensholt, H.H. 8
Burke, Edmund 1, 199
Butler, R.A., and prison building 5

Chilad, B.S. 51
Churchill, Winston 2
Coornhert, D.V. 88–9

Datir, R.N. 34, 48, 53 n.10
Dhagamwar, V. 53 n.14
Di Julio, J.J. 174
Downes, David 6, 9–10

Ekland-Olson, S. 174
Ellis, O.B. 173–4, 176–7, 180–2, 185
Estelle, 178, 184–5

Geurts, A.C. 98
Gibson, C.S. 196–7
Gregory-Smith, Graham 24

Hewlings, David 7
Howard, John 1–2, 3, 10, 115; on
  administration 195; *An Account of the
  Principal Lazarettos in Europe* 196–7;
  on alcohol 178–9; biography
  188–200; on classification 177–8; on
cleanliness 13, 182, 194; as country
gentleman 191, 197; criticisms 195;
death and funeral 199–200; on
differentiation 194; early life and
education 188–9; in Europe 196,
197–8; evaluation 198–9; on health
and disease 13, 193–4, 199; as High
Sheriff of Bedfordshire 191–3;
marriages 189–91; and Netherlands
prison system 6, 90, 198; on
overcrowding 183; on prison
discipline 176; proposals for
national penitentiary 5; quoted 1,
69, 84; on staff 3, 174, 175–6, 185,
186; *The State of the Prisons* 69, 90,
170, 172, 186, 188, 194–6; visits
Maidstone Prison 13, 186; on work
179–81
Howard, John Jr 190–1, 197
Hurd, Douglas 16

Iyer, Krishna 51

Jenkins, Michael 7–8
Jester, Beauford 173

Kelk, C. 98, 99
Khan, M.Z. 51
Krumsiek, Herr 157
Kumar, S. 50–1

Lewin, Hugh 85 n.3

Martin, S.J. 174
Mathieson, Thomas 4
Mihalik, J. 85 n.3
Miller, Jerome 3, 8

202

# NAME INDEX

Mulla, A.N. 37, 51
Murray, Ken 7

Nayar, Kuldip 32–3, 50–1

Ortega, Daniel 127

Paterson, Alexander 175, 185
Perrie, Bill 7, 8
Peters, A.A.G. 98

Richardson, G. 37
Roberton, Alan 7

Schama, Simon 89, 93

Schoen, Ken 8
Scott, Sir Walter 188
Simmons, Lee 173
Singh, I. J. 50
Sinha, S. 40
Spieghel, 89
Srivastava, S.P. 50

Theroux, P. 23
Tulkens, Hans 8
Tyler, M. 50–1

Ward, D.A. 2
Wood, Frank 7

# SUBJECT INDEX

Lightning Source UK Ltd.
Milton Keynes UK
UKOW040609300312

189874UK00001B/3/A